放血療法

The Complete Guide To Chinese Medicine Bloodletting

Dean Mouscher

DISCLAIMER

Treatment using needles should only be done by appropriately trained and licensed practitioners.

The author has made every effort to ascertain that the information presented in this book is accurate. However, no warranties or guarantees, express or implied, are made. It is possible that there are errors both typographical and factual. Neither the author nor publisher assume any liability or responsibility for any loss, injury, or damage arising from or related to any use of the material contained herein. The treating practitioner, relying on his or her expertise and knowledge, alone is responsible for determining the best and safest treatment for his or her patient.

Copyright © 2018

Cover art and book design by Daria Lacy

All rights reserved. No part of this book may be reproduced or transmitted in any form or by any means, mechanical, electronic or otherwise, without express written permission from the author, except brief excerpts for purposes of review.

Your support of the author's rights is greatly appreciated.

ISBN 978-0-692-18102-7

Published by:
Crandon Publishing
Highland Park, IL
info@chinesebloodletting.com

www.chinesebloodletting.com

First edition

Acknowledgments

I am so grateful to those who helped me create this book. Without them it could not have been done.

I would first like to thank the late Master Tung for selflessly making possible the continuation of his work. To save his family's acupuncture tradition for posterity, Master Tung trained disciples and left us with a book. Without that, this great acupuncture tradition—previously never taught outside the Tung family—would be lost.

Thanks to Wei-Chieh Young, a senior disciple of Master Tung, for his prolific writing and teaching of Master Tung acupuncture and bloodletting.

Thanks to Chuan-Min Wang, another direct disciple of Master Tung, for generously and energetically sharing his first-hand knowledge through videos, seminars, a book, and personal communications, and for permission to quote him in this book.

Thanks to Brad Whisnant for generously sharing with me his experiences and knowledge of bloodletting.

Thanks to Susan Johnson, who generously teaches and keeps alive the Master Tung tradition of bloodletting.

Thanks to Kristen Horner Warren, who read through an early version, helped me understand how much more I needed to do, and created an outline around which this book took shape.

Thanks to Lorraine Wilcox who read through a later version, opened my eyes and helped me re-orient the book for a wider audience, and made so many helpful edits and comments.

Thanks to Laurie Lehey for looking through the book, giving me encouragement, and making excellent comments.

Thanks to my MD friend who prefers anonymity for all the technical and medical information she provided.

Thanks to Derek Talbot for his innovative explanation as to how bloodletting works.

Thanks to Sarah Roell for sharing her extensive experiences treating shingles patients both in China and the US.

Thanks to Deborah Bleecker for sharing her publishing experience and knowledge.

Thanks to Bret Shulman for allowing me to include the amazing experience he had with his son.

Thanks to Ted Zombolas for his advice and encouragement.

And last but not least, thanks to my family who put up with my absence and grumpiness as I struggled with this book.

For my patients, who taught me everything I know.

Note to readers:

Those who read this book from start to finish will note that certain important points amd illustrations are repeated throughout. Please forgive the repetition and understand that it is purposeful, as I would rather the information be found too often than missed by those who use this book as a reference.

Invitation to view pictures in color

The cost of printing in full color is prohibitive, which is why the pictures appear in black and white.

However, please go to www.chinesebloodletting.com to see all the important pictures in this book in full color.

Facebook group

Please join the Facebook group Chinese Medicine Bloodletting for up-to-date information and discussion of bloodletting.

Contents

Acknowledgments 3
Note to readers: 5
Invitation to view pictures in color online 5
Introduction 9
Chapter 1: The Power of Bloodletting 13
Chapter 2: Bloodletting—key concepts................................17
Chapter 3: Bloodletting and Western Medicine........................35
Chapter 4: Bloodletting safety 39
Chapter 5: Tools for Bloodletting...................................59
Chapter 6: Talking to patients about bloodletting...................69
Chapter 7: Bleeding the back 75
Chapter 8: Bleeding legs 111
Chapter 9: Bleeding ears 145
Chapter 10: Additional areas to bleed..............................151
Chapter 11: Clinical guide to bloodletting by indication 171
Chapter 12: My favorite conditions to treat with bloodletting......205
Chapter 13: Case studies 211
Appendix I—Supplies 239
Bibliography 242
Endnotes 243
Index 245

Introduction

When I finished acupuncture school in 2001, I wasn't all that confident in my clinical skills. So I ventured outside my TCM training and, on the advice of a teacher, took a seminar with Dr. Richard Tan.

What a revelation! I was blown away by how elegant it was, and how it allowed me to instantly relieve so many complaints—a quantum leap in effectiveness.

Spurred on by that success, I learned other microsystems as well. I studied Koryo Korean Hand Therapy, Nogier-style ear acupuncture, and scalp acupuncture with Dr. Yamamoto in Japan.

After a few more years in practice, I was pretty proficient in all those styles. I thought I was a pretty darned good acupuncturist—if I did say so myself!

About that time, Master Tung style was becoming all the rage. Acupuncturists the world over were raving about and trying to reproduce the great master's results.

I wanted to learn Master Tung style too, and bought a book by Weh-Chieh Young, one of Master Tung's senior apprentices. In the introduction, I came across a section entitled "How to recognize a qualified acupuncturist."

Qualified acupuncturist? Why, that was my middle name!!!

Young listed five requirements to be a qualified acupuncturist. With smug certainty that I would ace them all, I started to read.

Number 1 was "Fewer points selected." Yep, I was pretty spare with my needles. Number 2—"Careful selection of points." Yes again—no random needles in my clinic, each one had a purpose! Number 3—"Needling not applied to the diseased site." That made me three for three—I was a distal guy all the way. Number 4—"Instant results for emergency and painful cases." Absolutely—Dr. Tan had taught me how to make acupuncture work fast.

But Young's fifth and last qualification stopped me cold: "Bloodletting for protracted and complicated cases."

Bloodletting? Seriously?

"Blood stasis," continued Dr. Young, "occurs in protracted, difficult and odd diseases, for which bloodletting is the best way to solve the problem… If properly conducted, unimaginable effects can be seen… Master Tung was especially good at bloodletting with a three-edge needle. An ailment persistent for years or sharp pain would be cured in an instant; the effectiveness is really beyond imagination."

And then the coup de grace: "Any acupuncturist who is not familiar with bloodletting cannot be viewed as a proficient one."[1]

Ouch!!!

I had to admit that I knew nothing about bloodletting. Like most acupuncturists, I hadn't learned much about it in school—maybe we spent a few hours on it. What I *had* learned was purely theoretical—I had never done it and really didn't know enough to actually try it. What kind of needle would I use? How would I keep my patient from bleeding to death? I had no idea.

All I really knew is that you can bleed jing-well points to clear heat. And if you were crazy enough, you could bleed a vein at UB40—for what exactly, I wasn't sure.

But apparently I would have to learn. I wasn't about to spend the rest of my life as an unqualified acupuncturist!

Thus began the obsession that has consumed the past several years of my life—studying, experimenting, and learning all I could about the subject of bloodletting.

I studied bloodletting from the TCM angle, learning—among other things—that it is the original practice from which acupuncture evolved. I studied it from the Western medical and phlebotomy angles, learning what can go wrong and how to do it safely.

And most of all, I studied it from the Master Tung angle.

Master Tung, I discovered, bled some 30-40% of his patients, among them his toughest cases. Bloodletting was a routine, everyday practice in his clinic—and in large part responsible for his stellar clinical results.

Master Tung's system of bloodletting was intricate and highly developed, often bleeding points and areas unknown to TCM.

Fast forward to today. After having performed thousands of bloodlettings every year for many years now, I wonder how I ever practiced without it. I wonder how ANY acupuncturist practices without it, as it is so often the key to unlocking the most difficult, acute, stubborn problems. Every day I have clinical successes with bloodletting that would be out of reach without it.

Introduction

And I've made it my life's work to breathe new life into this ancient practice—to show acupuncturists how important bloodletting is, and how "doable" it is.

The reality of bloodletting is so different from what most acupuncturists imagine. My fondest hope is that this book will reset your conceptions about it. You will learn that contrary to what you may have thought, bloodletting is easy to do, quick, readily accepted by patients, painless, and safe. It is not limited to vague uses such as clearing heat but, rather, is the best treatment for so many common complaints—able to instantly relieve the most acute pain and stubborn conditions.

Chapter I

The Power of Bloodletting

Many years ago, a huge guy limped into my clinic with crippling sciatica, his face contorted in pain. Each step made him wince. It was torture to watch.

At that time I had never bled a patient, so I did my best acupuncture on him. But when he stood up and grimaced in agony, I knew I had failed.

I'd been thinking about bleeding, and wanted to bleed, and was terrified to bleed all at the same time. But this patient was in SO much pain, he was the perfect test case. It was now or never. So I had him lie face down. He was wearing shorts, which was convenient. The sciatica was in his left leg, so I looked at his left UB40 area.

And there—behind his knee—was the most incredible network of dark purple spider veins I had ever seen.

I didn't really have a proper bleeding needle—just some diabetic lancets. I also had some safety lancets—the single-use, spring-loaded ones. Nowadays I tell people you cannot use safety lancets to bleed spider veins because you cannot aim spring-loaded lancets precisely enough to hit those thin veins. Moreover, the lancets are too short. But back then I didn't know any better so I took a safety lancet, aimed as best I could, and pushed the button.

My heart was pounding—I was terrified. But by some miracle my safety lancet hit a bulls-eye, precisely piercing a spider vein in the middle of the web. Dark purple blood oozed out at a good clip. The blood was so dark it was almost black.

As I was saying a silent prayer that my patient wouldn't die right there on my table, he suddenly uttered the words that would change my practice and my life. "Oh-h-h-h" he said, "I don't know what you're doing but whatever it is, don't stop. That tightness is really coming off my thigh."

Really? So fast? So easy? Immediate, dramatic relief from the worst case of sciatica I had ever seen—just by releasing a bit of blood from behind his knee?

Twenty minutes later he walked—not limped—out of my clinic with some 90% relief. He hardly looked like the same person who had walked in—he was all smiles. I couldn't believe it. It was the healing magic I had always dreamt about. That was it. I was hooked.

Why I wrote this book

After that initial success, I was hungry to learn all I could about bloodletting. But detailed instruction was simply not available. What little information there was used procedures and instruments I would not use in my clinic, and that my patients would probably not accept.

It occurred to me that while bloodletting is an ancient art, it's the 21st century now and better, safer, and more painless instruments and techniques are readily available. There's no reason to limit ourselves to what acupuncturists used and did decades, centuries, and millennia ago. We can make bloodletting painless and acceptable to patients, while still reaping its incredible clinical benefits.

So I started experimenting with modern advancements such as safety lancets, which are painless—patients literally feel nothing. And disposable plastic cups, which eliminate the time-consuming process of sterilization while dramatically reducing the possibility of cross-contamination.

To establish safe guidelines I studied phlebotomy, the modern science of drawing blood—a highly developed discipline with a well-established safety record.

Over many years a new, updated approach evolved—a blend of ancient bloodletting wisdom and modern, painless procedures using up-to-date medical instruments and technology. Bloodletting this way is as easy for patients to accept as simple acupuncture, while losing none of its incredible clinical benefits.

Using modern instruments, procedures, and guidelines also takes bloodletting away from the fringes of acceptability and puts it squarely where it belongs—front and center as a mainstream acupuncture practice that is safe, painless, and will pass the scrutiny of even the most hard-nosed health inspector.

These procedures transform bloodletting from a major undertaking to be used only in the most dire cases to a simple procedure that can be safely and easily done every day. We can finally stop treating it like the black sheep of the TCM family and instead for what it is—possibly the most powerful healing practice in Chinese medicine.

So after many years and thousands of bloodlettings, I wrote this book. It is meant to be the bloodletting manual I wished I had when I started bleeding—a nuts-and-bolts guide to incorporating bloodletting into your practice.

The vast majority of this book is drawn from my personal experience performing bloodletting in my clinic over many years. There is little in this book I have not done myself. It is a contemporary approach to bloodletting that is easy to do, safe, and proven effective.

Chapter 2

Bloodletting—key concepts

Which side do you bleed?

In bloodletting, we ALWAYS bleed ipsilateral to the pain or symptoms, that is, on the same side. This is very consistent—I know of no exceptions.

Capillary bleeding vs. venous bleeding

In the next section we will talk about the three main areas for bloodletting—the ear apex, the back, and the legs.

But before we get to that, let's talk about an even broader classification. Specifically, all bloodletting can be divided into capillary bleeding and venous bleeding.

Capillary bleeding occurs when the skin is punctured in an area where there are no visible veins. A needle such as a diabetic lancet is used, and the puncture or punctures are very shallow—2mm or less—just into the dermis. When a diabetic pricks his or her finger to get a drop of blood to test for blood sugar, that's capillary bleeding.

In capillary bleeding, blood seeps from capillaries into the puncture and comes out slowly. The flow can be helped by squeezing or by a suction cup—wet-cupping is a form of capillary bleeding. When you remove an acupuncture needle, occasionally a droplet of blood oozes out—that also is capillary bleeding.

One of the major types of bleeding outlined in this book is bleeding points on the back, particularly the upper back. If you look at the backs of most people, there is nothing to see except skin—there are no visible veins. So bleeding the back in most cases is capillary bleeding too—you make a few shallow punctures into the skin, then encourage a little blood flow by cupping.

Another major type of bleeding outlined in this book is bleeding the apex of the ear. There too you will generally see no visible veins. You prick the skin with a diabetic lancet and squeeze out a little blood—this too is capillary bleeding.

Capillary bleeding is simple and safe. With a puncture depth no greater than 2 millimeters, little can go wrong. When you stop squeezing or remove the cup, bleeding generally stops quickly on its own, and can be stopped at any time with light pressure.

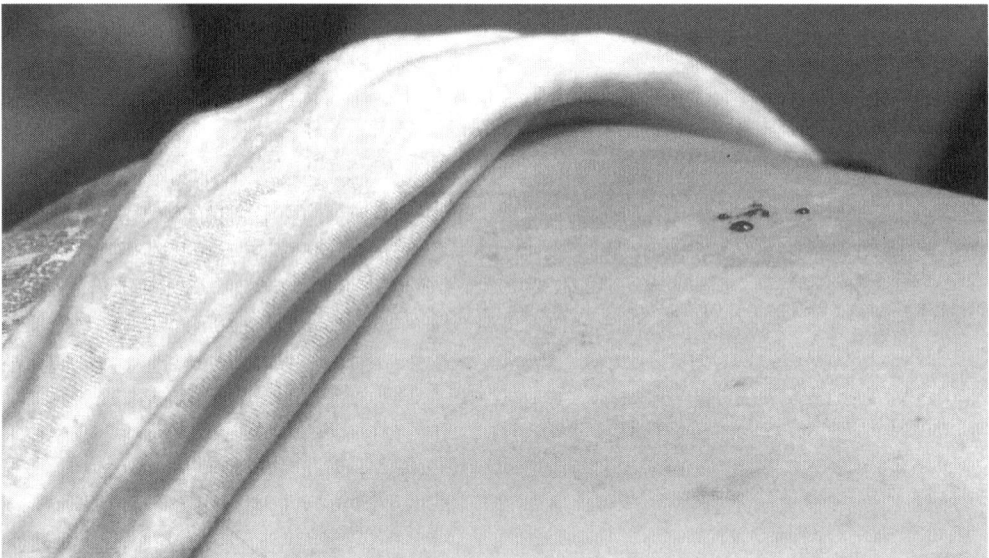

Fig. 2-1. Capillary bleeding on a patient's back. The back has been lanced 4 times using 4 separate safety lancets. The next step will be to apply a suction cup to help draw out blood. That is the reason for the cup in wet-cupping—without the cup, capillary bleeding yields little blood. *Full-color picture at www.chinesebloodletting.com.*

Bloodletting—key concepts

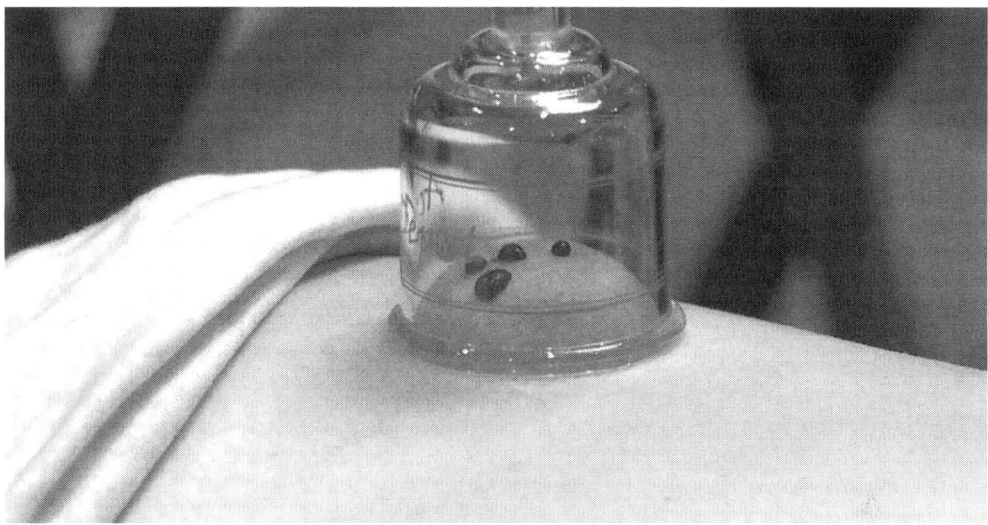

Fig. 2-2. Here the cup has been applied. You can see how the suction helps draw out blood during capillary bleeding. This is wet-cupping. *Full-color picture at www.chinesebloodletting.com.*

Venous bleeding is when a visible vein is punctured. Examples are veins in the crook of the elbow, such as those punctured for an IV or blood donation. Also—and more importantly for our purposes—venous bleeding is when we puncture a visible vein in the leg.

Venous bleeding is the same as "bleeding luo vessels" in TCM terms.

Venous bloodletting is also very safe—again, bleeding can be stopped at any time with gentle pressure. But it can require a bit more skill—and sometimes a bit more caution—than capillary bleeding.

Bleeding veins is only slightly more daunting than capillary bleeding, especially if—as recommended—you bleed the most superficial, darkest veins. More on this later.

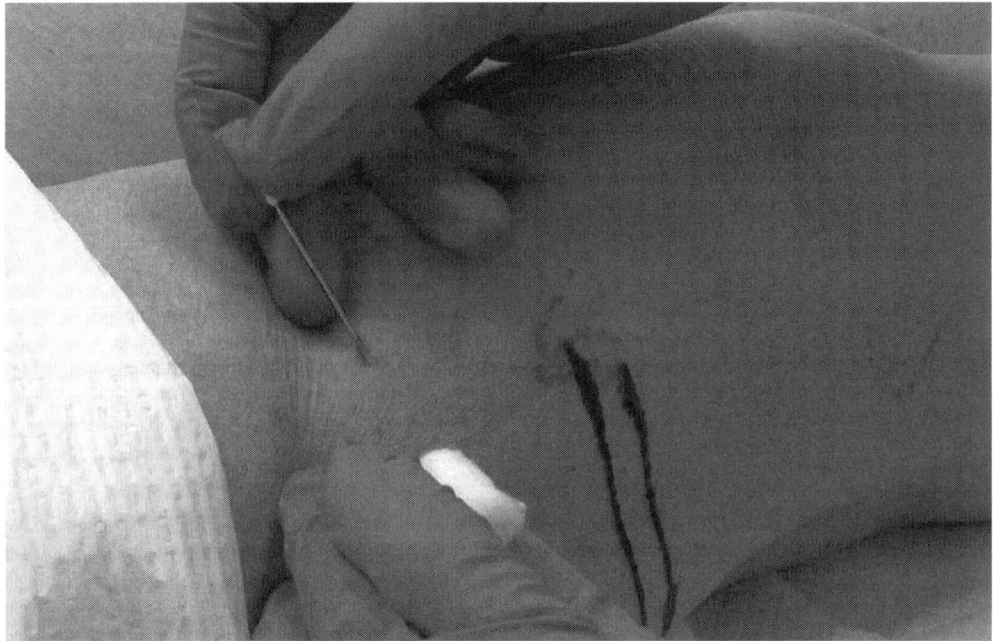

Fig. 2-3. Venous bleeding above the knee using a 1.5" 18 gauge hypodermic needle. Thumb and forefinger hold the top of the needle while the middle finger controls the tip. In venous bleeding, no cup is necessary. Note how dark the blood is. This is a sign of blood stasis and a welcome sign to the practitioner, as it is a good indication that blood stasis is being removed and that the procedure will be effective. *Full-color picture at www.chinesebloodletting.com.*

I will briefly mention Arterial bleeding, which occurs when an artery is punctured. We haven't mentioned arterial bleeding because in Chinese bloodletting we NEVER want to puncture an artery, as there is no therapeutic value in doing so.

Arterial blood is easy to recognize as it is bright red and under high pressure—it will squirt with each beat of the heart.

Arteries are easy to avoid but should you puncture one by accident, you can stop it with pressure on the puncture wound, maintained for at least 5-10 minutes, and dressed with a pressure bandage afterwards.

A pressure bandage is best done with a wad of gauze over the puncture, and pressure applied by a nonadherent bandage (a bandage that adheres only to itself such as Coban) around the limb. Pressure should be firm and snug but should not cut off circulation.

In Western medicine, phlebotomists frequently puncture arteries to get samples of arterial blood, which are required for certain blood tests. So if you accidentally puncture an artery it is—with rare exceptions—not catastrophic. More on arteries in a later chapter.

The three main areas to bleed

With the above in mind, let's turn our focus to the three main areas to bleed—the legs, the back, and the ear apex.

When I teach bloodletting seminars, I can see there is a lot of confusion about how to bleed these different parts of the body—what bleeding instruments and techniques to use where. Let's clarify things here, keeping in mind the distinction between venous bleeding and capillary bleeding.

Most of the confusion is in grasping the different nature of bleeding legs vs bleeding the back. So let's put aside bleeding the ear for now, and talk about those two types of bleeding—legs and back.

The main difference between bleeding the back and bleeding legs is that on the legs, there are usually visible veins. The veins may be obvious and dark—like purple spider veins—or they may be greenish and faint.

Either way, when you bleed legs, you are bleeding veins. You are using a bleeding needle—typically a hypodermic needle—to directly prick a vein and let it bleed.

On the back, however—with rare exceptions—there are no visible veins.

That difference—visible veins on the legs vs no visible veins on the back—means that bleeding legs and bleeding the back are different in important ways.

Bleeding legs

When you bleed legs—since you are bleeding visible veins—your EYES are your guide. You use your EYES to determine the exact point to prick. You are looking for the most obvious, darkest veins. Ideal veins to bleed are dark purple spider veins, as in Fig. 2-4 below.

Sometimes there are no such "perfect" veins on a patient's leg—in that case you have to find the most visible vein you can. But always when bleeding legs you are looking for—and pricking—veins.

Since you are bleeding veins and have to be precise, you cannot use a spring-loaded lancing device. They are simply not precise enough, and you cannot aim the needle with the exactness required. For bleeding legs—which means bleeding veins—you have to use a manual device. I use—and highly recommend—18 gauge or 20 gauge hypodermic needles.

Since you are bleeding a vein directly, the blood will flow on its own. There is no need to cup.

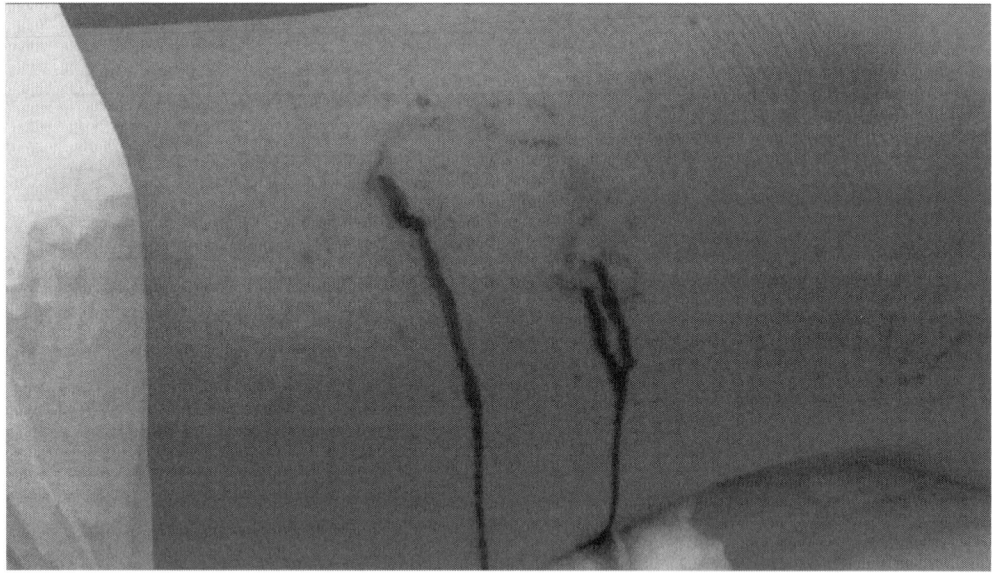

Fig. 2-4. Directly bleeding superficial "spider veins" in a patient's leg. The needle used was a 20 gauge hypodermic needle. Such veins are very superficial, and the needle is inserted just a few millimeters. Cupping is not necessary when bleeding veins directly. The amount of blood obtained was about a teaspoon (5 mL) from each prick. Full-color picture at www.chinesebloodletting.com.

To sum up:

- When bleeding legs, you are looking for veins and bleeding them directly.
- You need to use a more substantial needle than a diabetic lancet, which may not go deep enough. A hypodermic needle (just the needle, unattached to the syringe) is ideal.
- You don't palpate to find the exact spot to bleed, as you do on the back. Rather, your eyes are your guide. You are looking for visible

Bloodletting—key concepts

veins. Best are dark, prominent veins as in Fig. 2-4 above.
- Since you are bleeding veins directly, there is no need to cup. You will get an adequate amount of blood without cupping.

Detailed instructions for bleeding legs are in Chapter 8—Bleeding legs.

Bleeding the back

Let's turn to bleeding the back, where there are no visible veins. How do you know exactly where to bleed? By palpation.

For example, when bleeding the famous Tung area DT.07 for knee pain, you are palpating within a certain area, as shown in Fig. 2-5 below. If this is going to work, you will find one particular point to be the most tender to palpation. That is where you bleed.

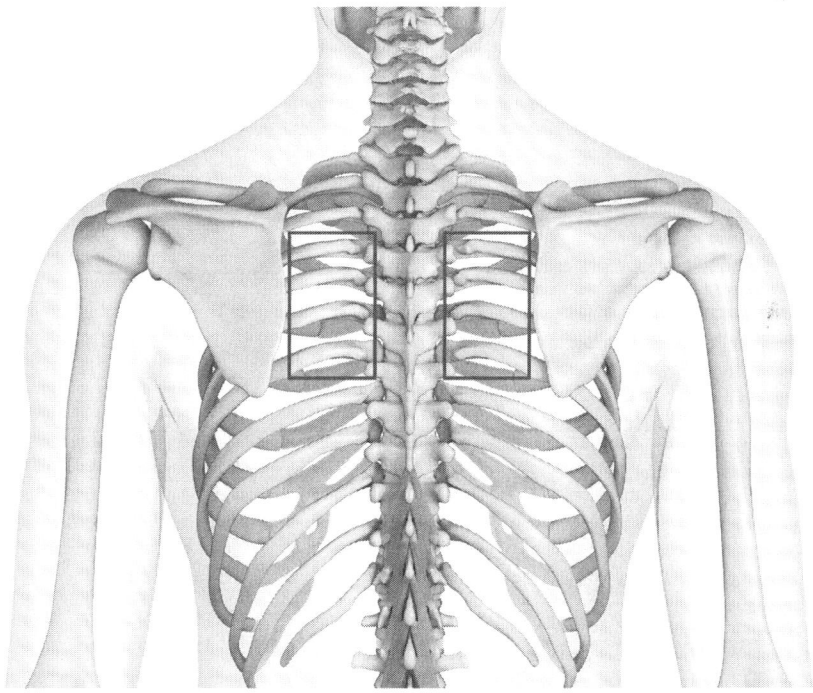

Fig. 2-5. Master Tung DT.07 area for knee pain

Due to the lack of visible veins, the type of bleeding done on the back is different. Instead of venous bleeding, it is capillary bleeding. You puncture the skin a few times with a lancet, and a little bit of blood oozes out.

In that case you have to use a cup to draw out more blood, otherwise you will barely get a drop. Again, that is the reason for the cup in wet-cupping.

You can use a hypodermic needle on the back as well, but that would be uncomfortable for your patient and I don't recommend it. For bleeding the back, the ideal tools are the 17 gauge McKesson safety lancets, sold under the brand name "Acti-Lance" outside of North America.

These safety lancets are safe to use even over the lungs, as the needle goes just 2mm deep. It is so sharp—and the spring action is so fast—that patients literally feel nothing, which makes it easy to wet-cup even your most needle-shy patients. Since the lancet can only be activated one time, there is zero possibility of accidental needlestick or cross-contamination.

I love these safety lancets. They make bleeding (wet-cupping) the back so easy, so comfortable for patients, and so safe. There are few contraindications to bleeding in this fashion—even older, weaker patients can generally be wet-cupped safely and comfortably.

I use four or five safety lancets for each cup. The punctures must be close together—within the 2 inch (50mm) diameter of the cup.

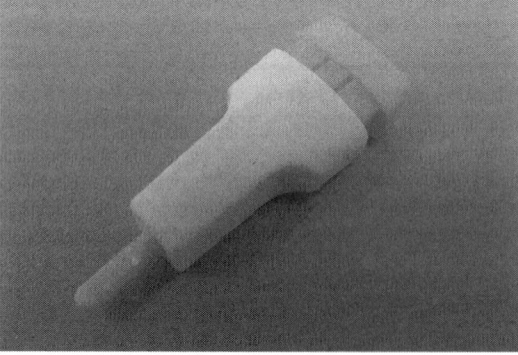

Fig. 2-6. McKesson 17 gauge safety lancets, sold under the name Acti-Lance outside of North America. Using these makes bleeding points on the back easy, safe, and painless.

So to sum up the differences between bleeding legs and bleeding the back: when bleeding legs you are bleeding a visible vein, your eyes are your final guide as to exactly where to prick, you use a manual instrument such as a hypodermic needle, and cupping is unnecessary.

When bleeding the back, however, there are typically no visible veins, nothing to see, so palpation is your final guide as to exactly where to bleed, you use

Bloodletting—key concepts

several spring-loaded single-use safety lancets, and you cup to get an adequate amount of blood.

To sum up bleeding the back:

- Since there are no visual clues to guide you when bleeding the back—no visible veins—you find the exact points to bleed by palpation. You are looking for points that are much more tender to palpation than the surrounding area.

- Since there are no visible veins to bleed, bleeding the back is capillary bleeding. Typically a diabetic lancet is used to make several shallow punctures in the skin at a point tender to palpation.

- Bleeding the back also requires wet cupping. You make the shallow punctures with diabetic lancets, then place a cup over the punctures to help draw out blood. Without the use of a cup, you will not obtain much blood.

Detailed instructions for bleeding the back are in Chapter 7—Bleeding the back.

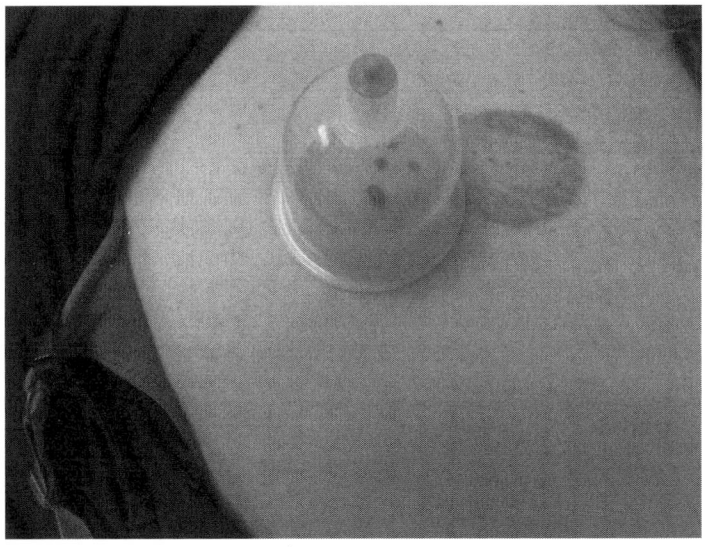

Fig. 2-7. Wet-cupping a patient's back after 4 painless, superficial pricks with spring-loaded safety lancets. You can see the adjacent wet-cupping mark from a few days earlier. *Full-color picture at www.chinesebloodletting.com.*

Bleeding the apex of the ear

This is also a type of capillary bleeding—although one can bleed the tiny venules as well.

Bleeding the ear is the easiest, fastest type of bleeding, and is easily accepted by patients. It takes just a minute or two, and patients don't even see what you are doing. Bruising rarely occurs—if it does it is mild—and patients don't see it. It is not painful and at most, patients feel a "mosquito bite."

Bleeding the ear apex is so easy—and so easily accepted by patients—that if there is any possibility of it being effective, I do it without a second thought. It literally takes just a few minutes.

What conditions will likely respond to bleeding ears? Pretty much any problem above T12 or so, particularly those with nerve involvement, and especially those of the head and upper limbs.

So any time a patient comes in with a headache, eye problems (including optic neuritis, stye, ptosis, and more), jaw pain, tooth pain, neck pain, nerve pain in the face (especially trigeminal neuralgia)—and anxiety/depression/insomnia—the first thing I do is bleed their ear.

In reality, you don't have to limit yourself to bleeding the ear apex only. I also often bleed a few additional points around the helix of the ear, as in Fig. 2-8 below. You can also look behind the ear—if there is a visible post-auricular vein, it can be bled as well.

Bloodletting—key concepts

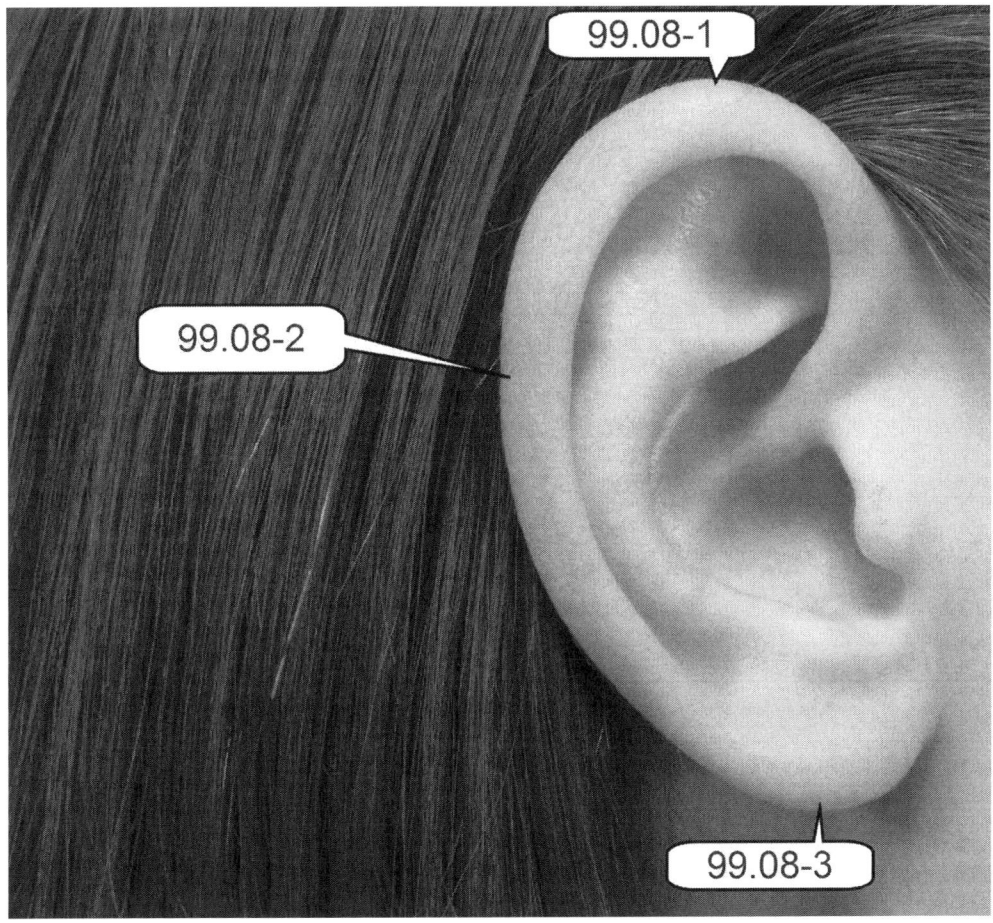

Fig. 2-8. In the Master Tung numbering system, 99.08-1 is the apex of the ear and the main point to bleed. I usually just bleed there when bleeding ears, but sometimes bleed an additional point or two on the helix between 99.08-1 and 99.08-2. *Full-color picture at www.chinesebloodletting.com.*

If the only thing you take away from having read this book is bloodletting the ear, you will still find your clinical results vastly enhanced, and obtain success with many patients and many complaints that were previously "out of reach." Detailed instructions are in Chapter 9—Bleeding ears.

Single-use, disposable needles and cups

Like acupuncture, bloodletting should be done exclusively with single-use, disposable needles.

For bleeding veins directly—such as visible veins in the legs—the best instrument to use is a hypodermic needle—the same ones used in hospitals and medical clinics.

As mentioned previously, to make a few shallow pricks in the skin for wet-cupping, the best instrument to use is a safety lancet. These are single-use, disposable, and painless.

I also highly recommend single-use, disposable cups. It is acceptable to use glass fire-cups for wet-cupping, but if you do they must be sterilized before re-using, as they have touched blood and are a bio-hazard. Remember that "sterile" means zero micro-organisms; sterilization is best accomplished with an autoclave.

Since the cups have touched blood, simple disinfection—reducing the number of micro-organisms by wiping or dipping in a disinfectant such as bleach—is not sufficient.

DongBang company in South Korea manufactures single-use, disposable cups for wet-cupping. They are inexpensive, and you will save a great deal of time—and markedly increase safety for yourself and your patients—by using them. Sources are in Appendix I—Supplies.

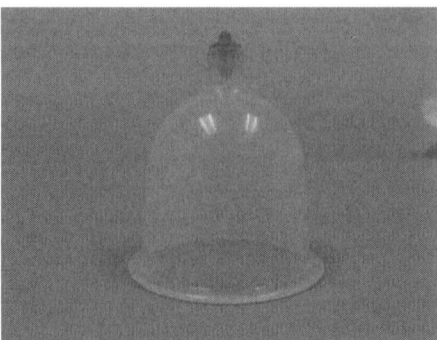

Fig. 2-9. Single-use, disposable cup made by DongBang. These come sterile from the factory, are inexpensive, and will save time and increase safety for you and your patients.

More is NOT necessarily better

You might guess that as I've become more experienced with bleeding, I've become more daring and aggressive. Actually, the opposite is true. Experience has proven that more blood is not necessarily better and that bloodletting is powerful, even when done conservatively and gently.

These days when I do bloodletting, I am more apt to go for the most superficial veins as opposed to deeper ones. That's because gentle and superficial is easier on me and easier on patients. And what I keep discovering over and over is that gentle bleeding with a small to moderate amount of blood is every bit as effective as aggressive bleeding, and more easily accepted by patients. And nothing is more important than creating a pleasant, stress-free experience for your patient. If they don't come back, you can't resolve their problem.

Blood stasis constitution

Some patients have a constitution that makes them prone to developing blood stasis. That means that a patient who has responded to bleeding for one condition is likely to benefit from it again for other, unrelated complaints that may develop in the future.

In other words, any patient who has responded to bloodletting in the past is likely to respond in the future, even if the new complaint is unrelated to the one that bloodletting "fixed." So in the future—whatever complaint this patient comes in with—bloodletting will be at the top of your list of therapeutic options.

Nerve conditions and nerve pain

Bloodletting has proven particularly effective for conditions with nerve involvement. Examples include radiating pain down the leg (as in sciatica), radiating pain down the arm, trigeminal neuralgia, optic neuritis, ptosis (droopy eyelid), nerve pain following surgery, and many more.

Any time a patient's complaint involves radiating pain or pain that seems to include nerve involvement or irritation, bloodletting should be the first thing you think of.

How does it work?

There are many explanations as to how bloodletting works using Western medical and anatomical concepts. I particularly like one proposed by a patient of mine who is a professor of anatomy at a medical school, and who himself experienced instant relief with bloodletting.

There are two venous circulatory systems, the deep venous system and the superficial venous system. The superficial veins are, for example, those you can see in the arms and legs. The deep veins lie beneath the fascia, which allows them to operate under higher pressures and handle higher volumes of blood—some 90% of blood is returned to the heart via the deep venous system while only about 10% is returned by the superficial system. The two systems are connected by perforating veins, so-called because they perforate the fascia.

The efficiency of blood flow in the deep veins is a question of venous pressure vs. tissue pressure. Venous pressure is the pressure pushing the blood through the veins back to the heart. Tissue pressure is the pressure exerted against the deep veins by the tissue surrounding them. So if there is an injury or inflammation, the swollen tissue can press against deep veins, impeding blood flow back to the heart.

The perforating veins offer an alternative route for blood flow back to the heart. If blood is having trouble flowing through the deep veins in a particular region of the body, blood can travel through the perforating veins to the superficial veins and then back to the heart.

A good example of this in Western medicine would be a patient presenting with "compartment syndrome," which occurs when the tissue pressure in an area exceeds the venous pressure, typically after an injury. The tissue swells and presses against the veins, impeding blood flow. Compartment syndrome is painful and sometimes debilitating. A similar situation can occur with an inflamed organ, nerve or joint.

With this in mind it is easy to see the meaning of "blood stasis." While Western medicine describes only certain limited cases of impaired blood flow in the deep veins such as DVT and compartment syndrome, Chinese medicine recognizes a broad phenomenon where increased tissue pressure in joints, muscles or organs can impede venous blood flow.

By letting blood at appropriate points, drawing blood off a superficial vein, you may also be drawing congestion off the muscle, nerve, artery or organ through the perforating veins. This removal of congestion can relieve pain and hasten the healing process.

Bloodletting and neurological reflex

A few years ago, I had a woman sit on a stool while I bled her ear apex. She was young and healthy and not at all nervous or anxious. But shortly after I pricked her ear and squeezed out a few drops of blood, she told me she felt "woozy"—then promptly fainted.

This incident was fresh in my mind recently—I had just written about fainting for this book (see page 44)—when I bled another young woman's ear, in this case for anxiety and sleeplessness. It was the second time I had bled her.

This time, when I was done, she turned to me with a somewhat puzzled look and said "both times you've done that, it relaxed me instantly. The first time I thought I was imagining it, but it just happened again. It's unmistakable, like something released. Is that possible? Could it really work so fast?"

And it struck me—although seemingly so different, could the reactions of the two young women to bleeding their ear be related? Could vasovagal syncope—the neurological reaction that caused the one woman to faint—be a variation of the reaction that caused the other woman to feel so relaxed?

Taking it a step further—could the healing power of bloodletting be partially due to a neurological reflex that occurs in response to loss of blood, in addition to any explanation involving blood flow dynamics?

My best guess would be yes. There are several reasons to believe a neurological reaction may be a part of bloodletting's healing power, as follows:

- Patients often say there is instantaneous improvement of symptoms—barely a drop comes out before they report relief.

- Vasovagal syncope—fainting—is said to involve a sudden lowering of blood pressure. And we know from experience how effectively bloodletting can relieve hypertension.

- Experience shows over and over that there is little correlation between the amount of blood that comes out and the amount of relief experienced. If the reason for bloodletting's effectiveness were purely the "fluid mechanics" of blood, one would expect that the amount of relief would be proportional to the amount of blood let.

This is speculation at this point of course—vasovagal syncope is poorly understood by Western medicine, while the healing power of bloodletting is as yet not even recognized.

How much blood do you need?

As mentioned earlier, one of the most important and surprising things about bloodletting is how little blood you need to make it work. The *Su Wen* specifies "a drop the size of a large bean"[2] and while you may get more, that is usually enough.

A great example: a 42 year old man came in with painful, bleeding hemorrhoids. I looked behind his knees and sure enough, he had dark veins in both UB40 areas. I pricked one of them and within seconds he looked at me and said "The pain is gone. Is that possible? Can it work that fast?" Not more than 1-2cc of blood had come out.

When he left, he commented again with amazement how great he felt. It is now more than a year later, and he has had no hemorrhoid pain or bleeding since.

So a small amount of blood can produce amazing results. But ultimately, the amount obtained depends on a few factors.

The type of bleeding tool and the practitioner's technique, of course, are part of the equation. But just as important—if not more important—is the patient's own constitution and physiology, and also the specific vein or area you puncture.

Some patients' blood—in certain veins—is under high pressure, and will gush forth or spurt the moment the prick is made. That is generally just a momentary phenomenon and not cause for alarm—the only danger as noted previously is that the practitioner may be startled and react suddenly, accidentally sticking him or herself. There's also the possibility that it could squirt in the practitioner's eye, so eye protection is a good idea. Always remind yourself mentally before pricking that a spurt may happen, although in my experience it occurs only once every 50-100 patients or fewer.

By the same token, the blood in some veins is under very low pressure. Even if you make a perfect stick with a good bloodletting needle, little or no blood will come out. If you don't get much blood from a puncture, it's not necessarily "your fault."

Phlebotomists recognize this phenomenon and are taught to choose veins by feel, not sight. They are looking for veins that feel full, and that rebound quickly from slight inward pressure. A phlebotomist told me that some veins are simply empty—if she inserts a needle into such a vein, the vacuum will simply cause the vein to collapse, and she will get no blood. You would need a tourniquet to use this technique however.

Sometimes, it's a matter of how well-hydrated the patient is. If they are dehydrated, the blood may not flow.

Another factor that varies from patient to patient is clotting time. Some patients' blood clots quickly, others' will ooze for quite awhile. If you have the time, it is always better to let the blood flow until it stops on its own. Otherwise there is the possibility that it will bleed later if, for example, the patient inadvertently removes the clot by ripping off the bandage too roughly.

Excessive bleeding of venous blood is almost never a consideration in practice because under normal circumstances, the blood flow will stop on its own and clot long before the amount of blood lost is a concern. In any case, it is easy to stop the flow by applying pressure with a clean cotton ball or gauze.

Many years ago I bought "Hemostatic Gauze" at a drugstore, which is described as "Gauze specially designed to turn into a gel that seals the wound to stop the bleeding." Several years and many thousands of bloodletting procedures later, the package sits in my treatment room unused. I would still advise having some on hand just in case, even though it is unlikely you will ever need it.

Chapter 3

Bloodletting and Western Medicine

Therapeutic phlebotomy

Phlebotomy is the western medical science of drawing blood. Mostly it is done for blood tests and blood donation.

But there is also a Western medical practice known as therapeutic phlebotomy which is, well, bloodletting! It's the same procedure as donating blood, except that the blood is discarded.

The two main conditions for which bloodletting—excuse me, therapeutic phlebotomy—is done in Western medicine are:

- Hemochromatosis
- Polycythemia

Hemochromatosis

Hemochromatosis is an inherited condition in which the body absorbs and stores excess amounts of iron. In some cases, it is severe enough to permanently damage vital organs.

The only treatment is therapeutic phlebotomy. Initially, a pint (about 470 milliliters) of blood is taken once or twice a week. Once iron levels have returned to normal, phlebotomy is done less often, typically every 2 to 4 months.

Polycythemia

Polycythemia vera is a type of blood cancer resulting in excess red blood cells.

One treatment for polycythemia vera is blood withdrawal, which "dilutes" the blood, resulting in a lower concentration of red blood cells.

Additional research on therapeutic phlebotomy

Reducing risk of heart attack

In Finland, the Kuopio Ischaemic Heart Disease Risk Factor Study[3] explored the correlation between blood donation and reduced risk of heart attack. It followed 2,862 men aged 42-60 for an average of 9 years, and compared the heart attack incidence of blood donors with non-donors. A donor was defined as someone who had donated blood in the 24 months preceding their entry into the study. Donors may or may not have donated blood after that.

The results were surprising. Of the non-blood-donors, 12.5% experienced an acute myocardial infarction (heart attack) during the study period of 1984 to 1995, while only 0.7% of the blood donors did. This shows an 88% reduced risk for blood donors—far more impressive than the reduction attributed to use of statins or—in all probability—any other known intervention.

An article in the medical journal "Perfusion" entitled "Cardiovascular benefits of phlebotomy" stated that:

```
"Renewed interest in the age-old concept of "bloodlet-
ting", a therapeutic approach practiced until as recently
as the 19th century, has been stimulated by the knowledge
that blood loss, such as following regular donation, is
associated with significant reductions in key hemorheolog-
ical variables, including whole blood viscosity (WBV) and
plasma viscosity… Reflecting these findings, blood donation
```

in males has shown significant drops in the incidence of cardiovascular events."[4]

Phlebotomy and metabolic syndrome

A 2012 randomized clinical trial on the effect of therapeutic phlebotomy on patients with metabolic syndrome (METS) concluded that "In patients with METS, phlebotomy, with consecutive reduction of body iron stores, lowered BP and resulted in improvements in markers of cardiovascular risk and glycemic control. Blood donation may have beneficial effects for blood donors with METS."[5]

"Current uses of phlebotomy therapy"

The journal "Hospital Practice" published an article titled "Current Uses of Phlebotomy Therapy" which states:

Despite its archaic origins and its general condemnation only a few decades ago, "bleeding" remains one of medicine's most important tools. In the conditions for which phlebotomy is indicated, the benefits may be profound and the risks small, compared with myelosuppressive and other toxic drugs. Its use for polycythemia vera and other diseases is discussed in detail.[6]

Chapter 4

Bloodletting safety

Bloodletting and phlebotomy

Phlebotomy is the drawing of blood for blood tests or donations, a common and safe procedure performed routinely in every hospital and medical clinic. Bloodletting has much in common with phlebotomy, and we can learn from it to help make bleeding safe for ourselves and our patients.

Phlebotomy guidelines are also well-established and accepted by local health authorities. By learning and following them, we can be certain to understand what health inspectors are looking for, and to pass any inspections that may arise.

Questions that come up frequently are: which tools and supplies need to be sterile (zero micro-organisms) and which ones are acceptable in a clean state? Do we need to don sterile gloves? Should we only be touching the puncture with sterile gauze, or is clean (but non-sterile) cotton wool acceptable?

We can safely answer these questions by examining the standards of phlebotomy established by the Clinical and Laboratory Standards Institute (CLSI) and the World Health Organization (WHO).

Phlebotomists are taught that there are just 3 sterile aspects of phlebotomy. These are:

- The alcohol swab used to clean the site to be punctured
- The needle itself

- The bandage

Protective gloves need not be sterile. The cotton or gauze used to wipe blood from the puncture or to apply pressure to the puncture need not be sterile either.

However, although not required, it is the policy of many clinics to use sterile gauze. Gauze is preferable to cotton because the fibers from a cotton ball can embed themselves in the clot and disturb it when the cotton ball is removed. Gauze has no such fibers, and the use of sterile gauze (as opposed to clean gauze) adds an extra layer of safety and hygiene. If a health inspector or public health nurse ever drops by, he or she will be positively impressed by your use of sterile gauze.

Unlike a phlebotomy clinic, I almost never artificially stop blood flow. When bloodletting, it is best to let the blood flow until it stops by itself. In fact, I squeeze around the puncture to encourage blood flow, and often wipe the puncture site repeatedly with an alcohol swab to prevent a clot from forming too quickly, and to keep blood flowing.

The exception is when I see a bruise forming at the puncture site. If I see "mounding" around the puncture site, I apply firm pressure for a minute or so (at least two minutes if the patient is taking anticoagulant drugs, or "blood thinners") to minimize the bruising, and for this I use sterile gauze. While non-sterile cotton or gauze is acceptable, a 2" x 2" (5cm x 5cm) square of sterile gauze is inexpensive, and I find comfort and satisfaction in knowing I am going "above and beyond" minimum safety standards.

And again—if you press on the puncture site with cotton wool, the tiny fibers become embedded in the clot as it forms. When you remove the cotton, those fibers may remove the clot and cause bleeding to re-commence. This is not a problem with gauze.

Clean Needle Technique and bloodletting

One needle per puncture

The CNT (Clean Needle Technique) manual includes a section on "Therapeutic blood withdrawal." These guidelines are less developed and complete than the phlebotomy standards, but you should be familiar with them.

The section contains "Critical Guidelines" and "Recommended Guidelines;" the former must be rigorously followed. The "Critical Guidelines" describe:

Bloodletting safety

- Hand sanitation
- Skin preparation
- Taking a thorough patient history including bleeding disorders, medication, supplement history
- The use of personal protective equipment (gloves)
- Inspecting the area to be bled for evidence of inflammation, lesion, infection, break in skin—do not bleed if present
- Requirement that lancets and needles are for single insertion only. Each site and each individual puncture requires a new lancet or needle.

All of these recommendations are common-sense except perhaps the last one, which I've bolded. Let's discuss it for a moment.

Once you have taken a bleeding needle out of its packaging, it may seem tempting to prick more than one point with it. However, that is a bad choice for several reasons—it is poor CNT for the patient's safety and just as important, it puts you at risk by increasing the probability of an accidental needlestick. Once you have made a puncture with a needle it is a biohazard and should be discarded immediately, not held and used again.

But an equally compelling reason to NEVER reuse a needle after a single insertion is that doing so is more painful for the patient.

The needles recommended in this book are razor-sharp and the first insertion is nearly painless. But that first insertion blunts the needle more than you might think, and the next insertion tears the patient's skin in a way that causes pain.

Take a look at the pictures following—on the left are virgin needles straight from the factory; on the right is the same needle after a single use.

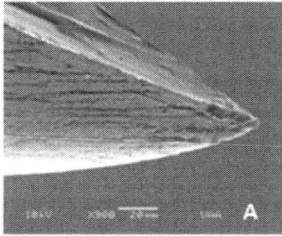 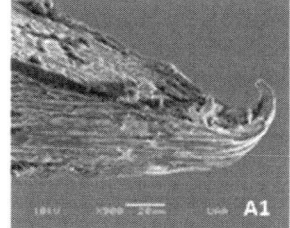

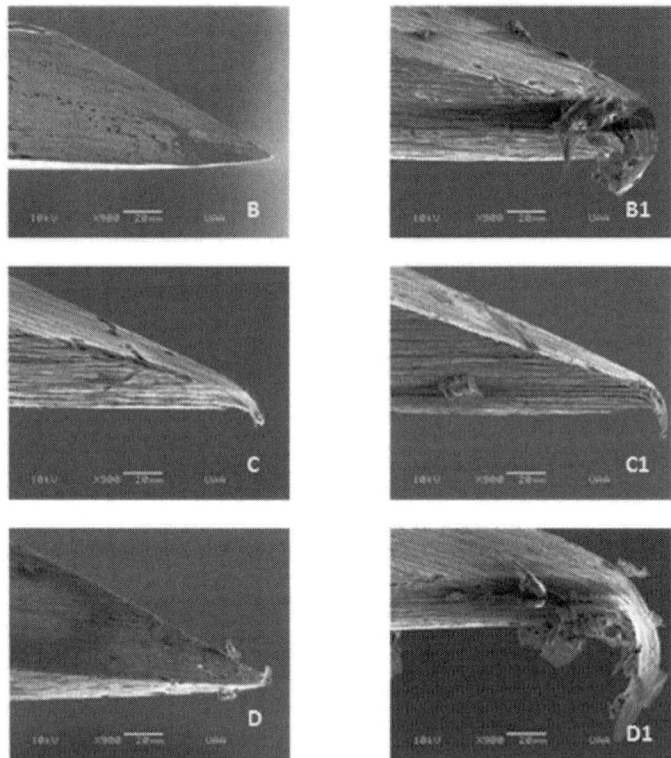

Fig. 4-1. Above pictures show the point of an unused needle on the left, and the same needle after one insertion on the right.

Is there a danger of taking too much blood?

Acupuncturists new to bloodletting are often concerned about letting too much blood. How much blood is enough, and how much is too much?

To put it in perspective, blood banks will allow virtually any reasonably healthy adult to donate blood. The amount taken is a pint—approximately 500 mL. That's two cups in the American measurement system, or 32 tablespoons.

Of the thousands of patients upon whom I have performed bloodletting, the maximum amount I have ever gotten—even without stopping the flow of blood myself—is approximately 100 mL, or 1/5 the amount of blood taken during standard blood donation.

What about anemia? Is it possible to cause anemia in a patient by letting too much blood?

Researchers have studied whether repeated blood draws from hospital patients can cause anemia. Their finding? It can occur, but only after a prolonged period of frequent blood draws. In fact, it was found to happen almost exclusively in intensive care units, and almost never in the rest of the hospital.[7]

In other words, non-ICU hospital patients—even those who have blood drawn frequently—are not at risk for anemia caused by phlebotomy.

Why is that? One large study found an average of 4.1 blood draws daily among ICU patients for a mean daily blood loss of 54 mL, and a mean total loss for ICU patients of 762mL during their hospital stay.[8] ICU patients also begin their stay depleted, and their impaired health can impede their ability to absorb iron and build hemoglobin.

Yet even among ICU patients, the authors found that total blood loss of less than 200mL is not clinically critical.[9] Again—after bleeding thousands of patients, the most blood I have ever obtained during a single session is about 100mL, and that is without artificially stopping the flow of blood.

Following is some information about hemoglobin levels in men and women.

13.5 -17.5 g/dl in men is considered normal

12.0 -15.5 g/dl in women is considered normal

Below 12.0 g/dl is considered mild anemia in women, but the anemia is not considered serious enough to consider a transfusion unless it goes below 8.0 g/dl.

For perspective on the impact of bloodletting on hemoglobin levels; a single blood draw of 15mL (one tablespoon) reduces hemoglobin by approximately 0.1 g/dl. A normal person eating a normal diet will absorb enough iron to rebuild that loss in about 2 days.[10]

So as you can see, the effect on hemoglobin levels of letting a small amount of blood is negligible.

Accidental needlestick

In truth, the biggest risk of bloodletting is not to the patient, but to the practitioner. Accidental needlestick and the resulting possibility of infection with a bloodborne pathogen is a real risk.

Unlike an acupuncture needle, a used bleeding needle is covered with the patient's blood or—if you are using a hypodermic needle—filled with the patient's blood. If you hold that used needle while dabbing blood or squeezing blood out, your hand can slip and an accidental needlestick can easily result.

Let's assume you are right-handed—If something unexpected happens (such as blood initially spurting), your left hand holding cotton or gauze may by reflex suddenly come over to cover the flow, accidentally coming into contact with the needle still held in the right hand.

The most dangerous time during bloodletting with a hypodermic needle is the time between the moment you prick the patient and the moment the needle goes into the sharps container. Make that time as brief as possible. Get in the habit of discarding the needle into a sharps container the moment you have pricked a vein. Then you are safe.

I suffered an accidental needlestick many years ago. It was so fast, I'm not even sure how it happened. My patient was a blood donor and the wife of a physician, and assured me at the time there was no problem. Blood testing since shows I was not infected. I was lucky. Still, it was a terrifying experience. Don't let it happen to you. Get in the habit of immediately pulling your hand away and dropping the needle into a sharps container the moment you prick your patient. It should be one motion—prick and discard.

Adverse reactions

Fainting

Some patients are prone to having a vasovagal reaction when blood is drawn, causing them to feel faint or even lose consciousness. For that reason, phlebotomists are taught to assume that every patient may faint, and to always position them in such a way that fainting will not result in a fall or injury—either by seating them with sufficient support or by having them lie down.

Having never gone to phlebotomy school, I learned that lesson the hard way.

Bloodletting safety

For the first few years, when bleeding ear apices I would always seat the patient on a stool. This was quick and convenient—after bleeding one ear, I would have the patient swivel 180 degrees and bleed the other ear.

It never occurred to me that the stool could be a problem. There were just a few drops of blood after all, which the patient didn't even see. What could go wrong?

After having bled several hundred patients that way without incident, one day I bled the ear of a new patient. She was young and healthy, and not nervous or frightened in the least.

But a few minutes after I pricked one ear, she told me she felt "woozy." Before I could react, she lost consciousness, fell off the stool, and ended up on the floor.

Fortunately she was unhurt, and regained consciousness without incident. We were both lucky. But as I later learned, not every case of fainting ends so well. There have been several lawsuits by phlebotomy patients who fainted while not properly seated or lying down and were injured. In one case, a patient broke his neck and was paralyzed.

Traditionally, the Chinese have patients stand to bleed UB40. Given what phlebotomy has taught us about vasovagal reactions and the possibility of fainting, I believe that practice is no longer acceptable. Always have your patients lie down when bleeding their legs, backs, or arms.

For bleeding ears, it may be more convenient to have them in a sitting position, but it should be done in a sturdy armchair that will prevent falling, even if the patient were to lose consciousness.

If the patient has a known history of fainting, always have them lie down, even when bleeding ears.

If a patient does faint, current guidelines recommend against using smelling salts as they can cause respiratory distress in asthmatic patients. Raise the patient's feet above heart level—they should regain consciousness quickly, in no more than a minute or two. After coming to, patients should stay in your office for at least 15 minutes, and should not drive for at least 30 minutes.

I also now have "instant cold packs" at the ready in my clinic in case a patient faints. Just take one and squeeze it, which causes chemicals inside the pack to mix together and produce instant cold. Place it on the back and sides of the patient's neck to revive them quickly.

To revive a patient who has fainted, Weh-Chieh Young recommends needling HT8 (22.10 in the Tung numbering system).[11] The classic TCM revival point is DU26, in the philtrum just below the nose.

Bruising

By far the most common adverse reaction to bloodletting is bruising. Capillary bleeding (such as wet-cupping) will rarely cause a bruise; they are generally associated with bleeding veins.

If the needle goes in too far and comes out the other side of the vein, this, of course, will cause bruising. But even if the practitioner does everything perfectly, in some patients blood will extravasate into surrounding tissue and cause a bruise.

You can see when a bruise is beginning to form by the greenish "halo" that surrounds the puncture site. Sometimes—especially when bleeding a vein in the cubital fossa—you will even see a small "mound" begin to form around the puncture.

When that happens, it is important to minimize the bruise by applying firm pressure for at least a minute and preferably two minutes (sometimes more if the patient is on blood thinners), to stop the subcutaneous bleeding and allow a clot to form internally at the vein. When you release pressure, observe the site for at least ten seconds to make sure bruise formation has stopped. Then you can apply a bandage.

The more superficial the vein you are bleeding, the less likely it is that a bruise will form. The purple spider veins are the most superficial, so when you bleed those, the formation of a bruise is unlikely. If you are bleeding a green, faint, deeper vein, bruising becomes more probable.

Bloodletting safety

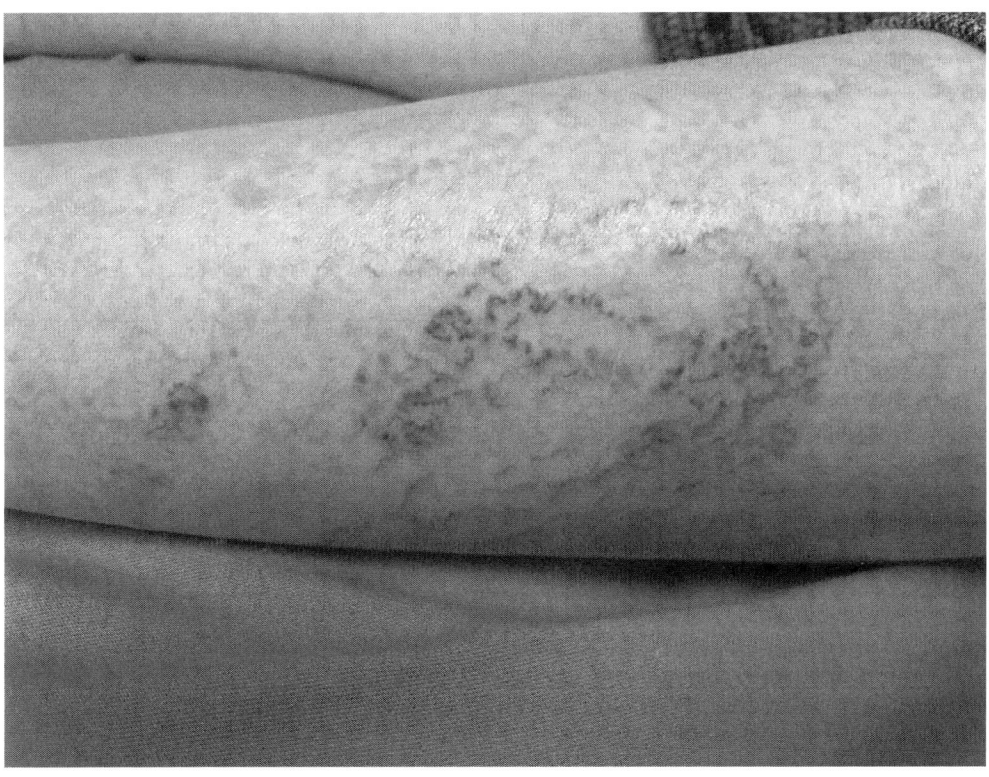

Fig. 4-2. Bleeding dark, superficial veins such as these is unlikely to result in bruising. *Full-color picture at www.chinesebloodletting.com.*

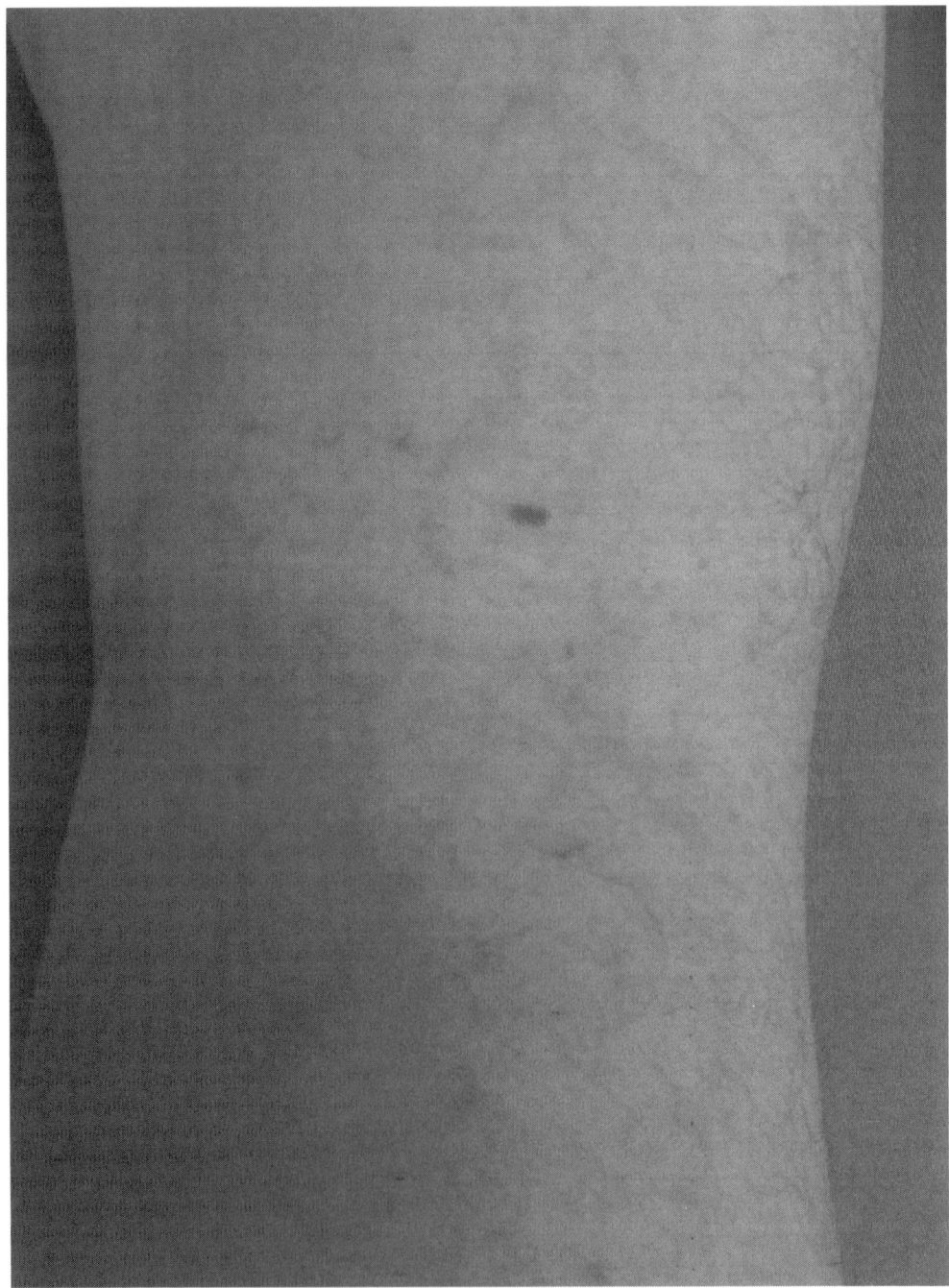

Fig. 4-3. Bleeding faint, greenish veins such as those pictured above is more likely to produce a bruise. Should you see one forming, simply apply pressure long enough for clotting to occur at the vein—approximately 2 minutes in most cases. When you

release pressure, observe the site for at least ten seconds more to make sure that subcutaneous bleeding (bruise formation) has stopped. *Full-color picture at www.chinesebloodletting.com.*

Should it look as though the patient will bruise, it is important to warn them. Simply tell them "It looks like this is going to bruise a bit, that's normal, it's just a bruise and will go away." Patients accept a little bruising if they expect it and know it is not a cause for concern.

If you don't warn them however, they may be shocked to see the bruise and think you did something wrong. In that case, you may get a phone call or an earful at the next appointment. Always let patients know when bruising may occur and it will not be an issue.

Contraindications and cautions

First, do no harm

In the following section, I have tried to give balanced information to help practitioners understand the risks of bleeding patients with certain conditions, so that they may make an informed decision as to when to bleed and when not to.

However, no text can take into account all possible variables. In the end it is your patient, your decision, and your responsibility. Use your judgment and be conservative—if in doubt, don't bleed until you have enough information to be satisfied it is safe to do so.

Poorly-controlled diabetes

Patients with poorly-controlled diabetes have impaired ability to heal, especially in the lower extremities. Such patients require extra caution. If a patient has advanced or poorly-controlled diabetes and/or neuropathy in the lower extremities, I am hesitant to bleed there, especially below the knees. If I do bleed their lower extremities, I will take the extra precaution of cleaning the skin with povidone iodine (Betadine) or other strong disinfectant before puncturing.

For these patients, it is safer to bleed their trunk and/or their ears. See Chapter 7—Bleeding the back, and Chapter 9—Bleeding ears.

How do you know if their diabetes is well-controlled? Most diabetics take frequent blood sugar readings—often every morning. Ask them what their reading is typically—if they average below 105 or so, then their diabetes is well-controlled and their risk of complications is low.

Advanced age

Older patients often have blood stasis issues, and can be significantly helped by bloodletting. I often bleed patients over 80 years of age, but am cautious when doing so—especially patients with paper-thin skin or purpura (purple blotches on their skin), an indication of fragile blood vessels.

The following example illustrates why. I had a female patient who was 87 years old. She was in reasonably good health for her age, but had excruciating pain in one shoulder that I could not successfully treat with acupuncture. Despite the purple discoloration in her leg and paper-thin skin—and perhaps against my better judgment as I was so anxious to help relieve the pain in her shoulder—I bled her ipsilateral lower leg.

She had many purple spider veins in the lateral lower leg to choose from, and I pierced one with a hypodermic needle. Immediately upon withdrawing the needle, blood began flowing freely out of the vein. Unfortunately it did NOT flow out of the puncture in her skin but, rather, spread in a rapidly-growing purple blotch under her skin.

The proper reaction would have been to apply firm pressure to the puncture and hold it for at least two minutes. That would have immediately stopped the blood flow and left her with just a small bruise.

However, I was new to bleeding at the time and didn't know what to do. By the time I thought to apply pressure to the puncture to stop the flow from the vein, the blotch covered a large area and looked awful.

She was nice about it, but I felt terrible. There was no lasting harm—within several weeks her body had absorbed the blood and no trace of the incident remained. Essentially, it was just a bruise. That will never happen if you simply remember to apply pressure.

It's also a good idea to use your judgment and, if in doubt, don't bleed veins. If it is a borderline case, you could consider limiting your bleeding to the back and ears (capillary bleeding) rather than the legs (venous bleeding), as this is safer and easier on the patient.

Anticoagulant drugs

A frequent question is: can you bleed patients who are on anticoagulant drugs, (blood thinners)?

You can generally feel safe performing *capillary* bleeding on such patients, as such bleeding is just from a few shallow punctures into the dermis. Capillary bleeding is not difficult to stop.

So the question is really "can you perform *venous* bleeding on a patient on blood thinners." In other words, can you prick a vein directly?

First, let's be clear what it means in practical terms if a patient is on blood thinners. Their blood will still clot, it just may take longer. In some rare cases it may take a lot longer.

The practical implication of delayed clotting is that you will have to apply firm pressure on the puncture for longer than usual—as long as it takes for a clot to form. As long as you apply pressure, the bleeding will stop. If a clot has not formed, the bleeding will resume when pressure is removed, but will stop again when pressure is applied.

So the answer to the question "can I bleed patients on blood thinners" depends to a large extent on how much time you have, and how much care you are willing to take. If you have sufficient time and patience, it can generally be done.

The concern is not really uncontrolled bleeding out, as bleeding out is easy to see and by applying firm pressure long enough, you can always stop the blood flow (although extreme cases may take time). You can also use a product such as hemostatic gauze to stop bleeding quickly (see Appendix I—Supplies on page 239).

The greater concern is subcutaneous bleeding. Sometimes blood will continue seeping from the vein but, rather than flow out of the puncture, it will extravasate into surrounding tissue, causing a hematoma, or bruise. If the patient is on blood thinners, this can continue for some time, resulting in a large bruise such as the one pictured in Fig. 4-4 below.

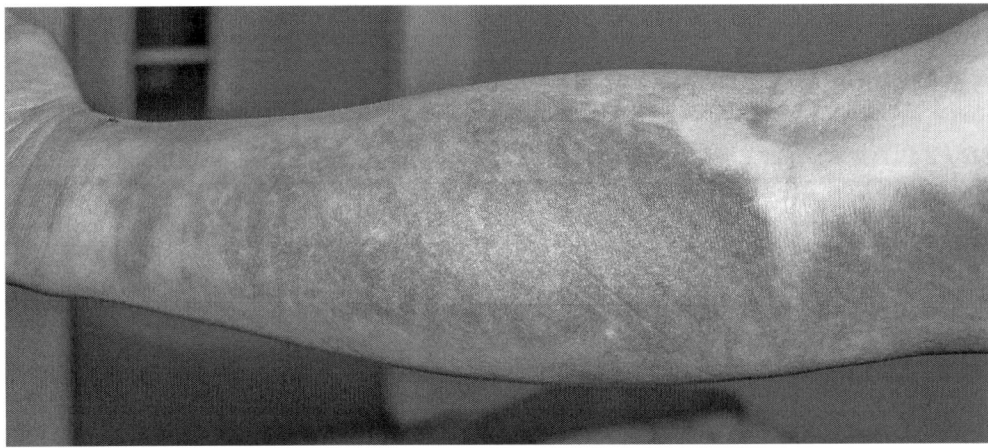

Fig. 4-4. By following proper procedure, bruising such as this can be prevented. *Full-color picture at www.chinesebloodletting.com.*

Besides being unsightly, in rare cases prolonged bleeding under the skin can result in compartment syndrome, exerting pressure on nerves and causing nerve damage.

This is easy to prevent. You need only apply firm pressure to the puncture for several minutes until hemostasis (blood clotting) occurs at the vein.

If you know the patient is on blood thinners, it is good practice to apply pressure to each puncture for a good two minutes or longer. When you release pressure, observe the site for at least ten seconds to make sure the bruise is not continuing to form—i.e., to make sure that subcutaneous bleeding has stopped.

It is also a good idea to ask questions beforehand to get a sense of how much the drugs affect clotting time. Does the patient notice that it takes a long time to stop bleeding if they cut themselves?

As a general rule, I prefer to bleed thin, superficial veins rather than deep veins in patients on blood thinners. Thin, dark, superficial veins are less likely to bruise.

While I personally have not had a problem bleeding patients on blood thinners, I have heard stories from colleagues of rare occurrences where bleeding took a long time to stop when bleeding veins. Always have on hand a product such as hemostatic gauze that will stop bleeding in such cases (please see "Appendix I—supplies" on page 239).

Bleeding disorders

Like anticoagulant drugs, bleeding disorders affect clotting time. Hemophilia is the worst bleeding disorder, and is of course an absolute contraindication to bloodletting.

It is generally possible to bleed patients with mild bleeding disorders such as Von Willebrand's Type 1. The advice and cautions in the above section, "Anticoagulant drugs," apply.

If you are familiar with the patient's bleeding disorder and know it to be mild, then you may consider bloodletting, with the understanding that clotting may take extra time. You will also want to favor bleeding the most superficial veins, and to do so conservatively.

If you are not familiar with the patient's bleeding disorder or are not sure, the wisest choice is to avoid bloodletting altogether.

Purpura

Some patients, especially elderly ones, have purple "blotches" on their skin. This is called purpura.

There are many possible causes—among them are anticoagulant drugs, platelet disorders, coagulant disorders and more.

Whatever the cause, purpura is an indication of vascular fragility and a reason for caution. I would avoid bleeding anyone with purpura unless I felt it was absolutely necessary in order to address their complaint. Even then, I would bleed minimally and only the most superficial veins, and only if I had sufficient time to be certain the subcutaneous bleeding had stopped before I let them go.

Pregnant patients

A frequent question is—can you perform bloodletting on pregnant women?

The answer you will find almost everywhere is no, don't bleed pregnant women. That's the easy answer and the safe one too—don't perform bloodletting on pregnant women and you will never face the legal consequences of doing so. In this litigious world, that may be reason enough to avoid it.

But what if the ONLY consideration is the good of the patient and child? Should you do it then? Is it safe?

One of the few authoritative discussions on the subject is in the book *Japanese Acupuncture, A Clinical Guide* by Stephen Birch and Junko Ida. It contains a chapter on Japanese bloodletting as developed and practiced by Drs. Kudo and Maruyama, two physicians who have practiced bloodletting extensively and written several books about it.

"Much of the content of these books focused on studies of the nature of blood stasis and scientific experiments to explore the physiological effects of bloodletting," write Birch and Ida. "Juxtaposed with this scientific data was a considerable amount of clinical data, enough to write a book on the subject."

So if anyone is qualified to opine on the safety of bloodletting pregnant women, these two physicians would be it.

And here is what they say: "Usually any acupuncture technique or treatment on a pregnant woman should be more gentle and at a lower dosage than usual. Certain acupoints or areas of the body are contraindicated for needling. There are similar restrictions or precautions that need to be followed when using bloodletting techniques.

"Pregnant women tend to be very sensitive to treatment, so it is important to avoid certain areas and techniques and to carefully regulate the dose of bloodletting. Bloodletting with cupping and bloodletting of the jing points are both considered to be too strong for pregnant women, and better avoided. If bloodletting is to be used, it should be only by the squeezing method, either after piercing a vascular spider or applying small cuts to a skin area. It is better to avoid the low back area.

"Usually bloodletting is only used when varicose veins need to be addressed as a common complication of pregnancy. In such instances, small vascular spiders are selected on the legs for bloodletting and moxa cones are used afterwards.

"Provided that you avoid the use of bloodletting with cupping, that you avoid bloodletting the jing points, and that you follow the guidelines for treatment on the legs only, bloodletting on pregnant women should be safe. If the patient has other health issues, such as difficulty walking or a history of miscarriages, it is better not to use the bloodletting techniques when treating a pregnant woman."[12]

I would add that women with gestational diabetes prick their fingers all day long, and nobody suggests it is a risk for miscarriage. Doctors order blood draws of pregnant women with no thought that it puts the pregnancy at risk.

So bleeding ear apices, or taking a few drops of blood from the back of the neck (Tung bleeding area DT.03, see page 81) for nausea, seems very safe. If it prevents the woman from taking a drug for her headache or nausea, then the risk/reward calculation would further favor gentle bloodletting.

Sciatica is another common discomfort during pregnancy; pricking the upper-back Tung bleeding area DT.08-DT.09 (see page 84) is often effective and should be safe as well. If you would like to be extra cautious, you can skip the cupping and just squeeze out a little blood.

Authors Birch and Ida specifically state that bleeding spider veins on the legs of pregnant women suffering from varicose veins is a common and safe practice in their experience. See "Varicose veins" on page 208.

Mastectomy with lymph node removal

Many patients who have had a mastectomy have also had lymph nodes removed from the ipsilateral armpit. Removal of axillary lymph nodes affects the drainage of lymphatic fluid, and is generally thought to make the limb more susceptible to infection, and make any infection more difficult to treat.

Axillary lymph node removal also creates the possibility of the limb becoming edematous (lymphedema), and increases the risk for blood clots in the veins of the armpit.

For all these reasons, women who have had their axillary lymph nodes removed are typically warned that for the rest of their lives they should avoid needlesticks or IVs in that arm, to avoid blood pressure measurements on that arm, to take extra care to avoid insect bites in that arm, and many more such precautions.

An opposing view was expressed to me by a medical doctor who practices both acupuncture and bloodletting. She told me that she would not hesitate to bleed ipsilateral lymphedema—assuming the usual sterile conditions of course—and believes it would help.

Since conventional wisdom calls for avoiding needlesticks in that arm, however, I would treat axillary lymph node removal as an absolute contraindication for acupuncture or bloodletting in the affected arm UNLESS you have the express permission of the patient's physician to needle there.

The question may be moot, however, because bleeding the arm itself is probably not necessary, as bleeding the ipsilateral ear of such patients is highly effective and is not contraindicated.

Bleeding varicose veins directly

Varicose veins are ropey, protruding veins such as those circled in Fig. 4-5 below. You never bleed those directly. You will get more blood than you want, because the valves in those veins are not functioning and the veins are engorged with blood. Further, such bleeding has no therapeutic value, and will likely make the swelling worse, not better.

You can and should treat varicose veins by bleeding the dark, flat veins on the same leg. More on this later.

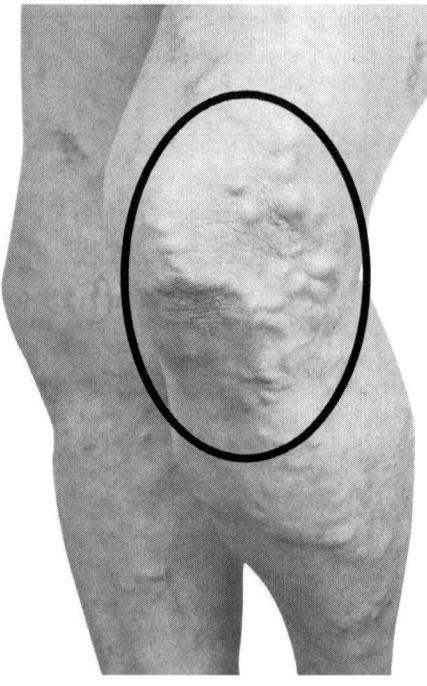

Fig. 4-5. Avoid bleeding varicose veins such as these. *Full-color picture at www.chinesebloodletting.com.*

Avoiding arteries

In Chinese therapeutic bloodletting we NEVER want to puncture an artery, as there is no therapeutic value in doing so.

Arterial blood is easy to recognize as it is bright red and under high pressure—it will squirt with each beat of the heart.

Arteries are easy to avoid but should you puncture one by accident, it is not a catastrophe. In Western medicine, phlebotomists frequently puncture arteries to get samples of arterial blood, which is required for certain blood tests. You can stop the bleeding with pressure on the puncture wound, maintained for

5-10 minutes or as long as it takes for the blood to clot sufficiently, followed by a pressure dressing.

Disposing of items contaminated with blood

Sharps, of course, must be disposed of in a sharps container. But what about cotton, gauze, and other items that are not sharp but have come into contact with blood?

World Health Organization (WHO) venipuncture guidelines state that items that would not release a drop of blood if squeezed may be double-bagged in appropriate plastic bags and discarded in general waste. However, you must check local regulations, which have final authority.

When disposing of blood that has gathered in a cup during wet-cupping, you must let it be absorbed by sufficient cotton or paper towels or other absorbent material so that it would not release a drop if squeezed. Some jurisdictions allow blood to be flushed down the toilet, as sewage systems are designed to handle biological waste.

What if you can't control the bleeding?

This is the nightmare scenario imagined by many novice bleeders, but it is not realistic. The bleeding is not from a chainsaw mishap, but from a tiny puncture made with a medical-grade instrument.

Bleeding will stop the moment you apply firm pressure. And unless your patient has a severe bleeding disorder such as hemophilia, a clot will form if pressure is applied for long enough. That is true even of patients on blood thinners who—as noted earlier—are more at risk from subcutaneous hemorrhage (hematomas, or bruising) than from bleeding out. (Note that pressure applied long enough will stop hematomas from forming as well).

Still, you should have on hand a product that will stop bleeding quickly. You will probably never need it, but you should always be prepared for the worst.

Many hemostatic products are available on the internet or in drugstores. They go under names such as hemostatic gauze, WoundSeal Powder, hemostatic sponges, and many more. Please see "Appendix I—Supplies" on page 239.

Chapter 5

Tools for Bloodletting

Needles and tools for capillary bleeding (the back, ear apex, fingers)

Safety lancets (ideal for wet-cupping)

Safety lancets are single-use, disposable units such as the one pictured in Fig. 5-1 below.

Within the unit is the steel lancet itself and a spring-loaded mechanism. It can only be activated one time, so cross-contamination is impossible. The needles are so sharp, and the action so quick, that they are virtually painless—the patient usually feels nothing.

These are ideal for bleeding the back—wet-cupping. My preferred needle width for these is 17 gauge. They are sold under the brand name McKesson in North America, and Acti-Lance elsewhere in the world.

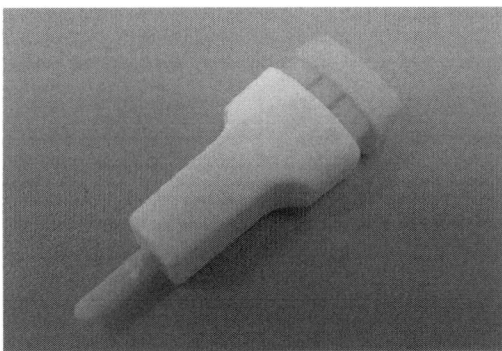

Fig. 5-1. McKesson 17g safety lancet, sold under the name Acti-Lance outside North America

I cannot say enough about how great these are for wet-cupping, and what a significant improvement they are over 3-edge needles for that purpose. Not only are they painless, they go just 2mm deep and so they can be used anywhere on the back with safely.

With 3-edge needles, wet-cupping the back used to be an ordeal. Using safety lancets, it is easier on the patient—and safer—than simple acupuncture.

These are also good for bleeding jing-well points. They can be used for bleeding ears as well. The only caution when bleeding ears is that if you have limited time, it might be better to use a 21 gauge manual lancet, as shown below. Using those, the quantity of blood is less, and the bleeding is faster to stop.

Manual lancets (ideal for bleeding ear apex)

For bleeding the apex of the ear, you can also use the 17 gauge safety lancets mentioned in the previous section. But for my purposes, these work a little TOO well. You get an adequate amount of blood all right, but it can take several minutes of applying pressure with a q-tip or gauze for the bleeding to stop completely. That is a long time in a busy practice.

That's why I prefer to use 21 gauge manual diabetic lancets for bleeding ears. I find these give just the right balance—you can get enough blood by squeezing it out drop by drop, but when you stop squeezing, the blood flow is usually easy to stop.

I don't always keep squeezing out blood until it stops on its own, as that could take a long time. Rather, I generally try to squeeze out 5-20 drops, then stop the flow and move on. I do this by holding a q-tip or gauze on the puncture site until the flow stops.

When bleeding ear apices, I first pinch up a bit of skin to avoid needling the cartilage. Not that needling the cartilage would be so terrible, but the gentler the better.

You cannot buy 21 gauge lancets in a drugstore—usually the largest-diameter lancet they sell is 26 gauge (the higher the gauge, the finer the needle). You will need to order 21g lancets online. The brand I most often use is EZ-Lets.

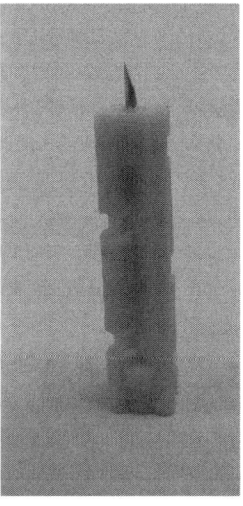

Fig. 5-2. EZ-Lets 21 gauge manual lancet

Cups

The modern, safe way to perform wet-cupping is with single-use, disposable plastic cups. DongBang company of South Korea manufactures such cups. They are inexpensive, save you time, and keep your patients safe from cross-contamination with blood-borne pathogens. See Appendix I for sources.

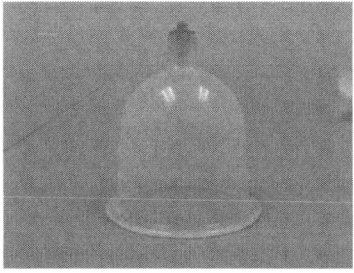

Fig. 5-3. DongBang single-use disposable cup. Use these for wet-cupping, and you can be certain that you are providing your patients with the highest level of protection from cross-contamination with blood-borne pathogens.

A note about cup inserts

One can buy plastic inserts as pictured in Fig. 5-4 below, but you should not use them for wet-cupping. The extra layer of plastic between cup and skin makes the vacuum seal unreliable. Air can leak into the cup and when it does, suction will be lost and you will end up with blood everywhere.

Also, you are handling the cup with gloves that will sometimes have blood on them, so you still end up with blood on the outside of the cup. You will have to sterilize it, and there is no good way of doing so.

In any case, the advent of inexpensive disposable plastic cups has made the use of these inserts obsolete. If you use a plastic cup for bloodletting, best is to throw it out when you are done.

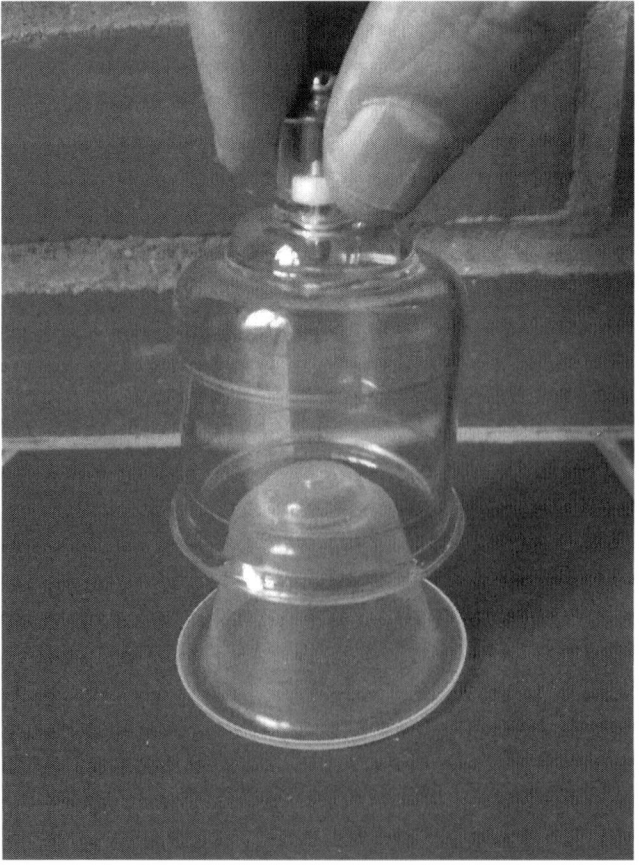

Fig. 5-4. For several reasons, the use of these cup inserts for bloodletting is not recommended.

Don't use reusable lancing devices!!!

These devices allow you to place a manual lancet inside. They are spring-loaded, and you can "cock" the device and lance over and over again.

The problem with these is that droplets of patients' blood can splatter on the device. Even a microscopic amount is enough to spread hepatitis B, which is highly contagious.

At least two outbreaks of hepatitis B have been traced to the use of such devices, one in Italy and one in California. [13] [14] They are fine for use at home, and can be re-used repeatedly by a single person. But they are not appropriate for use in a healthcare setting, or by more than one person. The safety lancets mentioned earlier are perfect for use in the clinic, as each is used just one time and the entire unit then discarded.

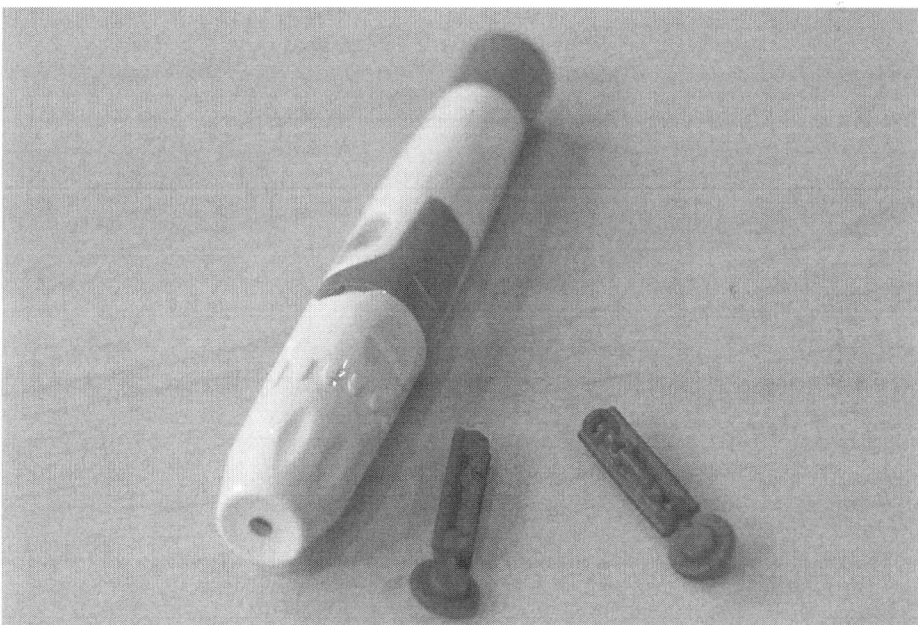

Fig. 5-5. Reusable lancing device. These are fine for home use by one person, but should never be used in a health care facility. Use single-use disposable safety lancets instead.

Needles for bleeding veins (as in the legs)

Hypodermic needles

After having experimented extensively with every type of needle and lancet available, I have settled on hypodermic needles (just the needle, not attached to a syringe) as the best instrument for bleeding veins.

The best sizes to use are 18 gauge and 20 gauge. The 20 gauge is a little gentler and goes in more easily; the 18 gauge gets a little more blood. For beginners I recommend 20 gauge needles, as they are a little easier to use and a little more painless. Get the 1.5" (approximately 33 mm) length; the 1" needles are too short.

I used to think that hypodermic needles are available only with a prescription, but every time I have ordered them online they were delivered without incident.

Hypodermic needles are razor-sharp and have a thin coating of medical silicone. They are generally not painful. They are also manufactured and sold by the same companies that supply hospitals, so you can be sure that they are made to the highest standards of safety and sterility.

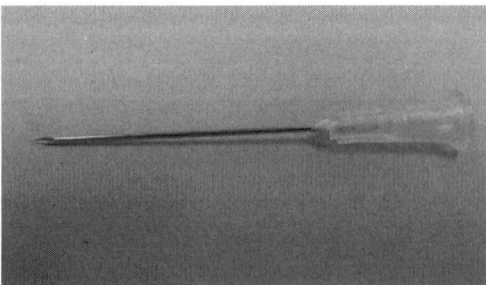

Fig. 5-5. McKesson 18 gauge hypodermic needle.

Piercing needles

Piercing needles are essentially cut-off hypodermic needles, and are mostly used by tattoo parlors for body piercing.

Although they are similar to hypodermic needles in form and sharpness, I prefer to use actual hypodermic needles.

Tools for Bloodletting

One reason is that hypodermic needles have a thin coating of medical silicone, while piercing needles do not. As a result, hypodermic needles are more comfortable for patients.

Also, the manufacturing origin of most piercing needles is murky and difficult to trace. Many come in plain boxes from China with no lot number or manufacturer name. Others are imported by American companies and have a brand name, but the importers I have checked with do not have paperwork indicating Good Manufacturing Certification or proof of ISO compliance. If ever there was a problem such as infection resulting from their use, you could possibly be liable for failure to do due diligence on the equipment used.

There is no such problem with hypodermic needles such as the McKesson or BD brands, which are the same as those found in hospitals and medical clinics.

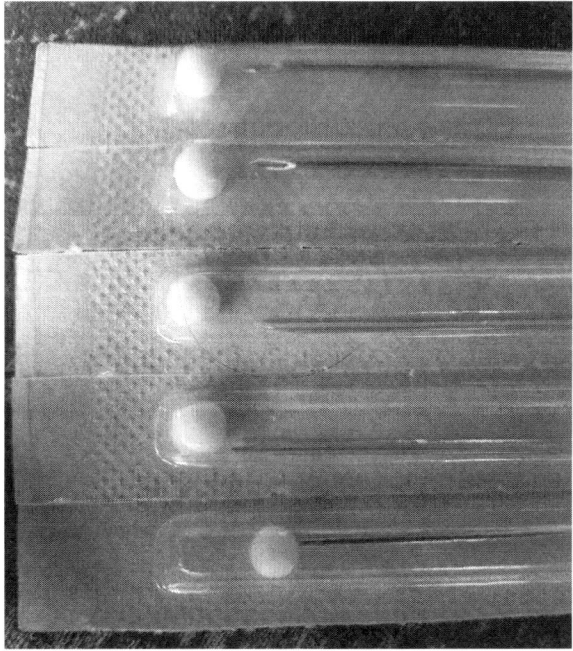

Fig. 5-6. Flat of piercing needles ordered through Amazon, and which arrived in a plain white unmarked box from China. As you can see, the styrofoam tips on 4 of the 5 needles came off during shipping, possibly compromising their sterility and rendering those needles unsafe to use. No documentation or certification is available regarding their manufacture or sterility, and it is impossible to trace where they were made or by whom. It is better to use name-brand hospital-grade hypodermic needles such as McKesson or BD.

Three-edge needles

You can buy sterilized single-use 3-edge needles, as shown in Fig. 5-7 below. The problem, however, is that they are not sharp and will cause excessive pain. Your patients will not like them, and neither will you. I recommend against their use.

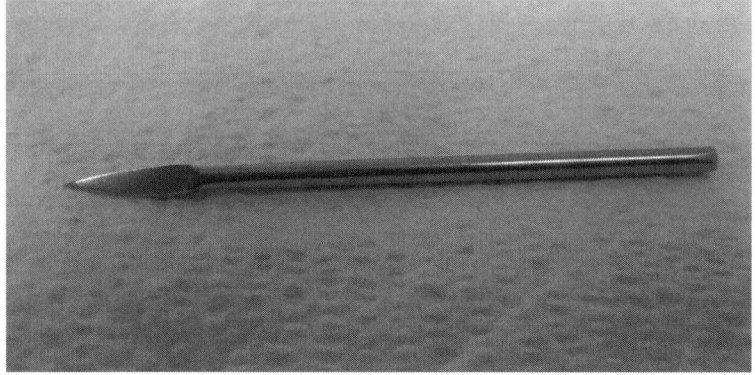

Fig. 5-7. Pre-sterilized 3-edge needle. These are dull when they come from the factory and are painful to use.

A small number of practitioners use traditional 3-edge needles that they hand-sharpen, sterilize, and re-use, but this is impractical for most. It also cannot be done in many states, which mandate the use of single-use, disposable needles.

Vein-finding technology

When bleeding veins, the veins are, for the most part, clearly visible. Occasionally, however, veins may be hard to find. In that case, a vein finder may help.

The best vein-finding devices use sophisticated technology and cost thousands of dollars. These are outside the budget of most acupuncturists, and they would be used so rarely that it would be difficult to justify such a large investment.

However, vein finders using simpler technology are available for a few hundred dollars. These devices are called "transilluminators," as they simply use LED light to shine through the skin and show the outline of hard-to-see veins.

Examples of such devices are the Venoscope II, and the Veinlite devices.

I have found these devices marginally effective, but somewhat useful with dark-skinned patients such as those of African and Indian descent. Dark skin makes veins harder to find, as there is less contrast between skin color and vein color.

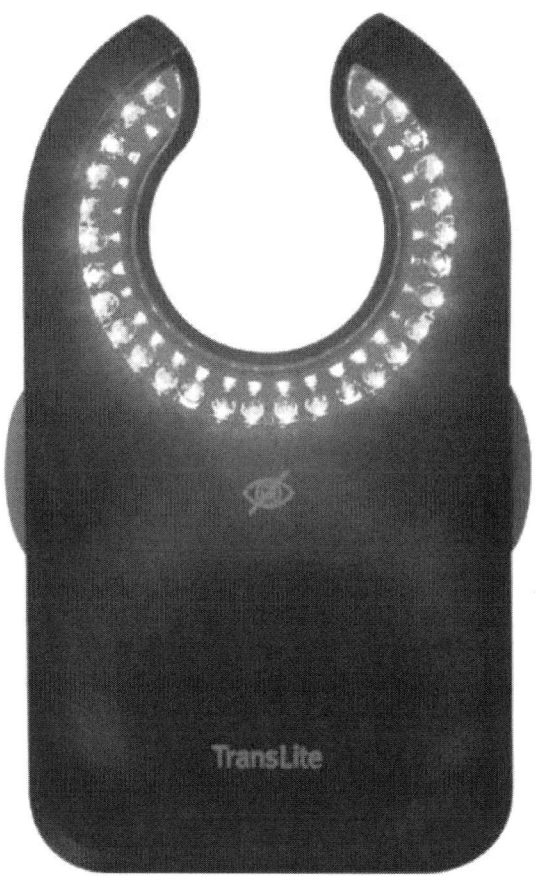

Fig. 5-8. Veinlite LED+

Chapter 6

Talking to patients about bloodletting

How to explain bloodletting to your patients

When I first started bloodletting, I loved the results but hated bringing it up with patients. I was afraid of frightening them and of making them think I was too "fringey." And in fact, the idea and the discussion did make some patients nervous and uncomfortable.

Today I bleed almost half my patients, and almost nobody objects or questions it. Bloodletting fits into my practice as comfortably as simple needling.

What changed? Two things really. Most important was my own confidence. Today when I decide to bleed someone, I KNOW it has a high probability of success, I KNOW it's safe and comfortable, and most importantly, I know that it's no big deal. The patient feels that confidence. They've come for the best treatment I can give them, and this is it.

The other thing that's changed is the words I choose. Instead of telling patients "I'm going to bleed you," I tell them "I'm going to try to get a few drops of blood." So rather than making it sound as if I'll be struggling to control the flow of blood, I emphasize how controlled the process will be, and how little blood I will obtain.

And really, the less said the better. If, for example, a patient comes in with a headache and I'm going to bleed their ear—the most common type of bleeding

I do—I'll simply say "I'm going to use a lancet—like the ones diabetics use to prick their fingers—and just poke the top of your ear and see if I can get a drop of blood. If I can, that usually takes pressure off and relieves the pain (or other symptom). Patients often feel relief immediately. So take good note of what it feels like at this moment because I'm going to ask you as soon as I'm done if there's any change. Is that okay?"

Most people are now curious and a little excited about the prospect of immediate pain relief and they say "You're the doc!" or "I'm here aren't I?" or words to that effect. Some patients ask if it will hurt, to which I respond "No more than a mosquito bite," which is generally true.

When bleeding veins in legs and arms, the needle I use is not literally a diabetic lancet, but close enough for our purposes when explaining the procedure to patients.

If a patient has more questions about how releasing a few drops of blood can ease their symptoms, I tell them that the veins we can see are just the superficial veins, but 90% of our veins are deep veins, and that congestion in the deep veins is often the cause of pain. I tell them that the deep veins are connected to the superficial veins, so if I can get a drop of blood from a superficial vein or even from capillaries in the skin, that can clear congestion and pressure in the deep veins, relieving pain and inflammation.

For additional information, see "How does it work?" on page 30 in Chapter 2—Bloodletting, key concepts.

Sometimes patients ask "What do you call this procedure?" Unless I know the patient is a huge fan of alternative medicine, I avoid the term "bloodletting." I tell them it's called "Fang xie" in Chinese, which means "removing blood stasis."

Sometimes I talk about how the first drops of blood are dark purple, almost black, because the blood has just been stagnant there, it's not been circulating properly so it is not oxygenated. After the first few drops the blood is red again, indicating that proper blood flow has been reestablished. Patients always respond well to that explanation, and if I perform bloodletting on them in the future they will often ask hopefully, "is it dark?"

Things to avoid saying

Again, the less said, the better. When bloodletting, the important thing is to avoid making a big deal of it. The more you talk about it, the more it sounds as though you have concerns, and the more it will make your patient uncomfortable.

When bleeding, don't give too many details. Don't tell the patient how their blood is spurting nicely, or how great the flow is. Some patients get squeamish at the sight of blood, so try to avoid letting them see any.

When bleeding the back, i.e. wet cupping, I may not even mention blood. The McKesson safety lancets I use are literally painless, the patient just hears and feels the click as the spring releases. If the patient asks what the click is, I tell them it's a lancet, as the procedure is more effective if I can get a few drops of blood. If they ask why, I tell them it relieves blood congestion and can take pressure off the nerve.

The patient feels the suction of the cup more than they feel the lancet, and therefore remembers the procedure as cupping, not bleeding.

Informed consent

Acupuncturists often ask me if I have patients sign a special informed consent before bloodletting. I do not. This is a personal decision for you to make of course, but in my opinion, doing so would call attention to the procedure and make it look dangerous. It's like telling the patient "I'm about to do something so risky that I need special permission from you." It's the opposite of what I want to convey, and of what I believe.

All patients sign an informed consent before doing acupuncture, and yours should reflect everything you might do, as well as the possible risks.

Establishing a baseline before bleeding

The first bleeding you do on a patient is diagnostic as well as therapeutic. If the patient responds at all, you know this is a blood stasis issue and that further bloodletting is warranted. If, however, the patient experiences no relief despite your best bloodletting, this is almost certainly not a blood stasis issue and no further bleeding is called for.

A good example is headaches. When a patient comes in with a headache, one of the first things I will do is bleed the ipsilateral ear apex, or both apices if the headache is bilateral or in the center. I am hoping of course that it will bring the patient some relief, but most importantly it will tell me if this is a blood stasis issue, and will help determine how I proceed with treating this patient in the future.

Before I start, I tell the patient that I will want to know if there is any small change after bleeding, so to please note well the intensity of the headache at this moment.

More often than not there is some level of improvement after bleeding, which confirms it's a blood stasis issue and tells me to look for additional sites to bleed. Typically I will then examine the ipsilateral leg or both legs if the pain is bilateral or in the center, and bleed where I see blood stasis, i.e. bleedable veins.

If there is no change in the headache after bleeding the ear, I will abandon the thought of bleeding for the time being, and look to see what other approach may be warranted.

What to say during the procedure

Not much needs to be said during bloodletting. If the patient is very interested in what I am doing, I may explain how bloodletting works, giving them more or fewer details depending on their level of interest.

But mostly, I treat this as a time to get to know the patient. It's a perfect time to ask them about their work, or their families, or to get more details about their health history and the specific complaint we are treating. In other words, a good time to just carry on a friendly conversation. Besides helping to establish rapport, friendly banter reassures the patient that everything is going well with the treatment, and that you are comfortable and at ease doing it.

A note about bruising

By far the most common adverse reaction to bloodletting is bruising. Capillary bleeding will rarely cause bruising; bruises are associated with bleeding veins, as in veins in the legs and the crook of the elbow

A bruise results when a vein is punctured and blood comes out but—rather than continuing out of the body—it spreads under the skin.

If the needle goes in too far and comes out the other side of the vein, this of course will bring about bruising. But even if the practitioner does everything perfectly, in some patients blood will extravasate into surrounding tissue and cause a bruise.

The more superficial the vein you are bleeding, the less likely it is that a bruise will form. The very purple spider veins are the most superficial so when you bleed those, a bruise is unlikely. If you are bleeding a green, faint, deeper vein, bruising becomes more probable.

You can see when a bruise is beginning to form by the greenish "halo" or "mound" that surrounds the puncture site. When that happens, you can greatly minimize the bruise by simply applying pressure for at least 2 minutes.

Why so long? The purpose of applying pressure is not to "squeeze out" blood from the tissue. Rather, it is to compress the vein so that hemostasis can occur beneath the skin, at the vein. Remember that a bruise results when blood leaks out of a vein and spreads under the skin. Pressure is applied to stop blood from flowing out of the vein long enough for a clot to form at the vein.

After you release pressure, observe the puncture site for at least ten more seconds to make sure that bleeding has stopped, and that a bruise is not continuing to form.

Once you see that a bruise has begun to form, it is important to warn the patient. I simply tell them "It looks like this is going to bruise a bit, that's normal, it's just a bruise and will go away." Patients accept a little bruising if they expect it and know that it is not a cause for concern.

If you don't warn them, however, they may be shocked to see the bruise and think you did something wrong. Always let patients know when bruising may occur.

Recommendations to your patient at the end of a session

If all you've done is to bleed a patient's ears, then nothing needs to be said about after-care. But if you've bled their back, leg, arm, or fingers, they will leave the clinic with a bandage over each puncture. Tell them to keep the area dry and to leave the bandage on for 4-6 hours, and tell them to be sure to remove it after that.

Follow-up

When a patient returns for their next treatment after a bloodletting session, always examine the puncture site to confirm all is well. The only time I ever found reason for concern was a patient with very fragile skin who had waited several days before removing the bandage on her back. The glue on the bandage had hardened and when she removed it, some of the outer layer of skin came off with it, leaving it looking like the aftermath of a blister that had popped and the loose skin removed.

I cleaned it thoroughly with povidone iodine (Betadine) after confirming that she was not allergic to iodine, covered it with sterile gauze, and explained the situation to her. I told her she would need someone to check on it daily for the next week or so to make sure it was not becoming infected. She lived with her mother and assured me she would have her look at it, keep the area clean, and check on it often. I carefully documented all that in her chart. When she came back a week later, it looked much better.

Chapter 7

Bleeding the back

The two main areas to bleed on the body (other than ear apex) are the back and the legs.

From a bloodletting perspective, the primary difference between these two areas is that on the legs, there are visible veins to bleed. On the backs of most people, however, there are no visible veins

That difference—visible veins on the legs vs no visible veins on the back—means that bleeding legs and bleeding the back are different in important ways. We will talk in detail about how to bleed veins in legs in a later chapter.

Since there are generally no visible veins on the back, how do you know exactly where to bleed? By palpation. Bleeding (wet-cupping) the back is always a matter of palpating within a certain zone and looking for a point that is extremely tender to palpation—much more tender than the surrounding area.

For example, one of the most common areas to bleed is the famous Tung area DT.07 for knee pain as shown in Fig. 7-1 below. If this is going to work, you will find one particular point to be the most tender to palpation. This is your target.

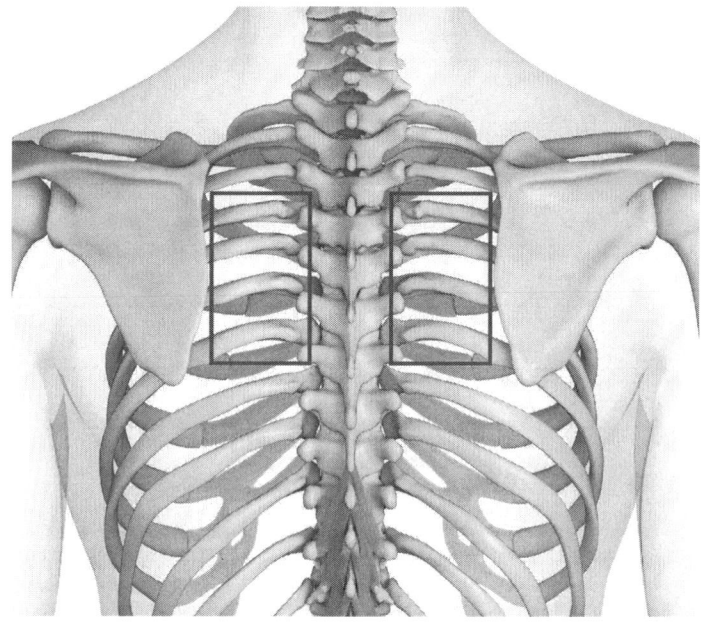

Fig. 7-1. DT.07. For severe degenerative knee pain, palpate within the box ipsilateral to the pain, and bleed (wet-cup) if you find a very tender spot.

Again, since there is no vein on the back, this is capillary bleeding. Puncture the skin a few times with a lancet, and a tiny bit of blood oozes out. You will have to use a cup to draw out blood in order to get more than a few drops.

You can use a hypodermic needle on the back as well, but that would be uncomfortable for your patient and I don't recommend it. For bleeding the back, I find the ideal bleeding tool is the 17 gauge McKesson safety lancets, sold under the brand name "Acti-Lance" outside of North America.

These safety lancets are safe to use even over the lungs, as the needle goes just 2mm deep. It is so sharp, and the spring action so fast, that patients literally feel nothing. Since the lancet can only be activated one time, there is zero possibility of accidental needlestick and cross-contamination.

I love these safety lancets. They make bleeding (wet-cupping) the back so easy, so comfortable for patients, and so safe. There is no barrier to doing it on even your queasiest and most needle-shy patients. There are few contraindications to bleeding the back in this manner—even older, weaker patients can generally be wet-cupped safely and comfortably.

I use four or five safety lancets for each point. The punctures must be close together—within the 2 inch (50mm) diameter of the cup. Then I place a cup over it to draw blood. I sincerely hope you discard the cup after use, as there is no way to adequately sterilize a plastic cup. Glass cups can be re-used, but must be sterilized first.

So to sum up—when bleeding the back there are typically no visible veins, nothing to see, so palpation is your final guide as to exactly where to bleed. You use several spring-loaded single-use safety lancets, and you have to cup to get an adequate amount of blood.

With rare exceptions, Master Tung never needled points on the back, he only bled them.

Master Tung system for bleeding the back

Master Tung was famous for his skill with a 3-edge needle. He performed bloodletting often—by many accounts, on some 30-40% of his patients. He bled all parts of the body, but his system of bleeding points on the back was particularly well-developed, with specific regions to bleed for specific conditions.

For bleeding points on the back, I personally favor and have had outstanding results with the Master Tung system. For that reason I am featuring it in this chapter, along with a few additional points.

Bleeding AREAS on the back vs. bleeding POINTS

In his only book, Master Tung depicted each bleeding area on the back by using several points. The idea was that the EXACT point to be bled on any particular patient could be at or near any of these discrete points. It was NOT meant to be a precise indication of exactly where to bleed.

This has unfortunately led to much misunderstanding over the years.

Take a look, for example, at Fig. 7-2 below, which shows the famous Master Tung "point" DT.07, also sometimes described as a "3-point unit."

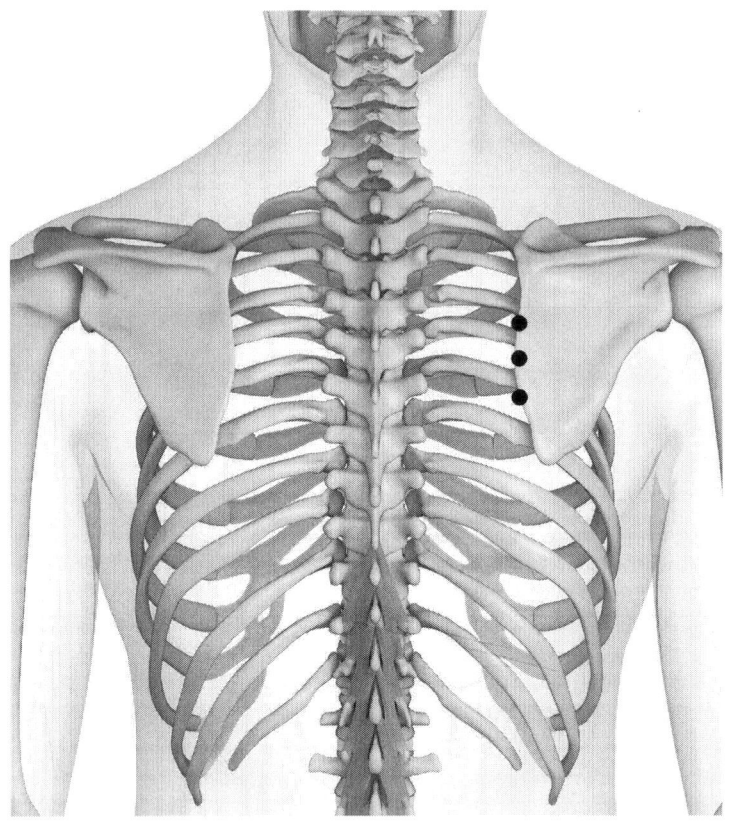

Fig. 7-2.

This illustration shows the 3 points of DT.07 as they are usually described—3 cun lateral to the spine, in the levels of T4, T5, and T6.

As a result, some have misunderstood that all 3 points should be bled. Others have suggested that the 3 points should be palpated and the most tender one bled.

However, after bleeding DT.07 for severe knee pain successfully on many hundreds of patients—probably close to a thousand times by now—it has become clear to me that DT.07 is best thought of as an area or zone rather than discrete points.

Fig. 7-3 below shows the approximate area in which I always find points to bleed for knee pain (when bleeding is appropriate and I find such points at all).

Bleeding the back

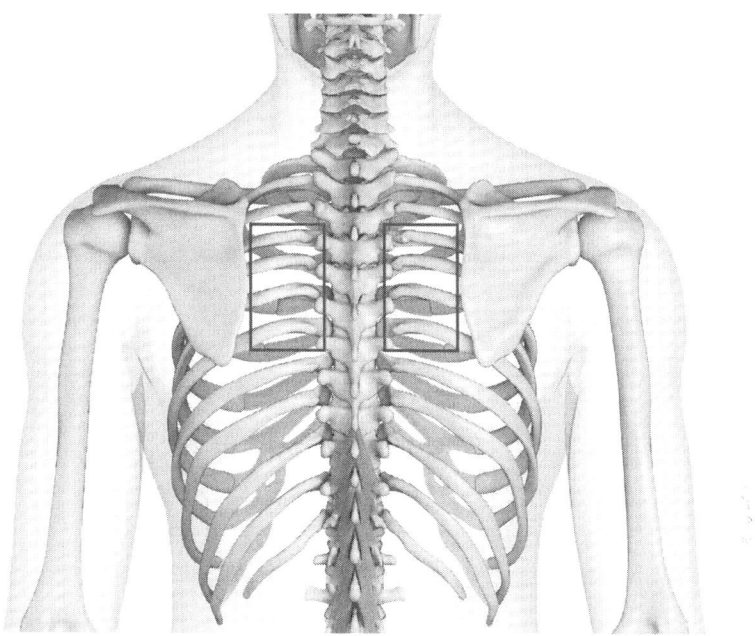

Fig. 7-3.

This is true of all the Master Tung back "points." Master Tung himself treated them as zones and not discrete points, and that is how I have elected to show most of them in this book.

I was happy to learn that no less an authority than Chuan-Min Wang—a disciple of Master Tung who worked under his direct tutelage in his Taiwan clinic—has essentially the same approach to interpreting Master Tung's instructions for bleeding the back.

Dr. Wang was kind enough to discuss with me his experiences in Master Tung's clinic in Taiwan. He emphasized repeatedly the importance of not following textbook point locations too literally, and of using one's own judgment and experience in the evaluation of each patient. "The map is not the territory" Dr. Wang told me. "Each patient is different."

In his book *Introduction to Tung's Acupuncture*, Dr. Wang had this to say about bleeding the back:

"...Master Tung employed bloodletting in a free and flexible manner. Just observe changes in the complexion of the trunk, palpate the muscle, tendon and bone, then you will know the location to prick...

"For example, let's consider [the point group] for knee pain DT.07. In 1973 Tung's textbook, [the points are] 3 cun away from T3-T5. Many practitioners use the exact measurements for these 3 points, but sometimes they cannot achieve good results.

"Personally I examine and palpate the channel after I have correctly located the points, and if there are changes such as tenderness, redness, or a rope-like sensation, I will needle the reactive spot instead of the exact location. If I do not find any reactive spots, I will not prick blood out in these areas. This is my approach for bloodletting performed on the trunk."[15]

Lateral upper back for severe itching and toxicity

DT.01 Fen Shi Zhang (Divided Branch upper point) and DT.02 Fen Zhi Xia (Divided Branch lower point)

The point DT.01 is located approximately at the bottom of the glenoid fossa, i.e. at the infraglenoid tubercle, one cun below the acromion of the scapula. Point DT.02 is located 1.5 cun below and .5 cun medial to DT.01.

For our purposes, we will describe this as an area, as pictured in Fig. 7-4 below.

Several sources point to DT.01 and DT.02 as points to be needled. However, others say it should be bled. In his book *Introduction to Tung's Acupuncture*, for example, Chuan-Min Wang—who as mentioned earlier worked alongside the Master in his clinic—describes bleeding DT.01 and DT.02 in a woman to cure a severe, itching rash in just two treatments. The rash was caused by exposure to hair dye.[16]

This area should be bled for severe itching anywhere in the body, such as that caused by poison oak or poison ivy. In Tung's acupuncture this is also known as an area where toxins accumulate, and bleeding this point helps to eliminate them from the body. This includes all kinds of toxins, from snakebites to drugs. It is also bled for excessive body odor and halitosis.

Palpate this area and wet-cup the most tender point or points.

Bleeding the back

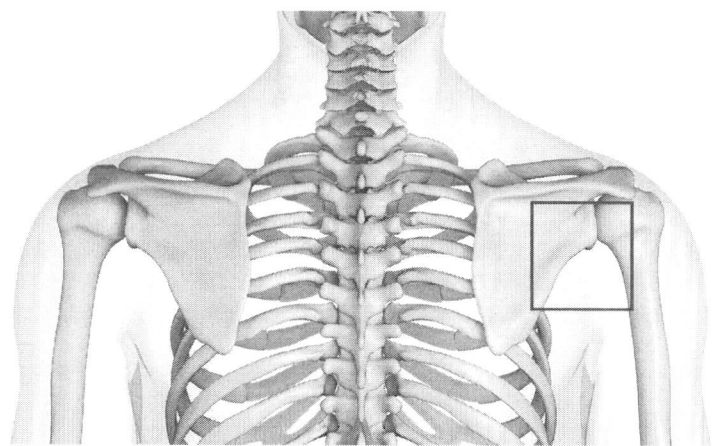

Fig. 7-4. DT.01-DT.02 area

Back of the neck for severe nausea

DT.03 Qi Xing (Seven Stars)

In some texts, the back of the neck is referred to as "point" DT.03. This is the go-to area to bleed for nausea and vomiting. Master Tung also used these for high fever and convulsions in infants.

DT.03 is often described as a "seven-point unit." The main points to bleed are DT.03-1, DT.03-2 and DT.03-3. DT.03-1 is located on the DU channel, just above the posterior hairline, in the depression just below the occipital protuberance. DT.03-2 is located one cun below that, and DT.03-3 is located one cun below DT.02.

There are another 4 points, located one cun to the left and right of DT.03-2, and one cun to the left and right of DT.03-3.

In reality, it makes more sense to think of this as a zone. But really, all you need is DT.03-1. For nausea, you can simply prick a few points at or near that point. Palpation is not necessary. Simply pinch up the skin and puncture with a few 17g McKesson safety lancets. Since it is above the hairline, cupping will not work and is not necessary. Simply squeezing out a few drops of blood is sufficient.

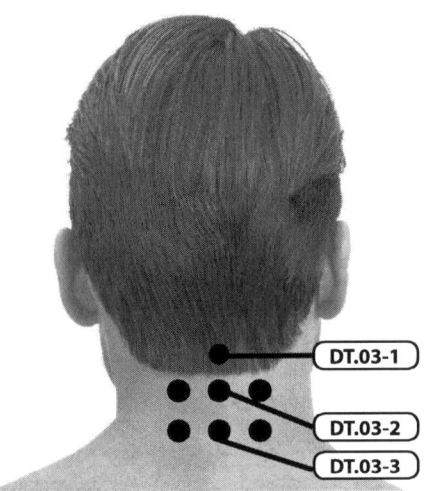

Fig. 7-5. DT.03. For nausea, just lance one or two times at or near DT.03-1 and squeeze out a few drops of blood.

Upper back

DT.04 Wu Ling (Five Mountain Ranges)

DT.04 comprises the entire upper and middle back. It is a combination of all the points in DT.07, DT.08, DT.09, DT.10, DT.12 and parts of additional groups.

Specifically, it comprises points on the spine from T1 to T12, points 3 cun lateral to the spine from T1 to T10, and points 6 cun lateral to the spine from T2 to T9—40 points in all.

DT.04 is such a large area that I have not found it as useful as other Master Tung point groups/areas, and in practice I do not use it.

DT.05 Shuang Feng (Double Phoenix) for pain, numbness and arteriosclerosis of hands and feet

DT.05 comprises an area approximately 1.5 cun lateral to the spine, from T3 to T9. Palpate for the most tender point, and wet-cup for pain, numbness, and arteriosclerosis of the four extremities.

Bleeding the back

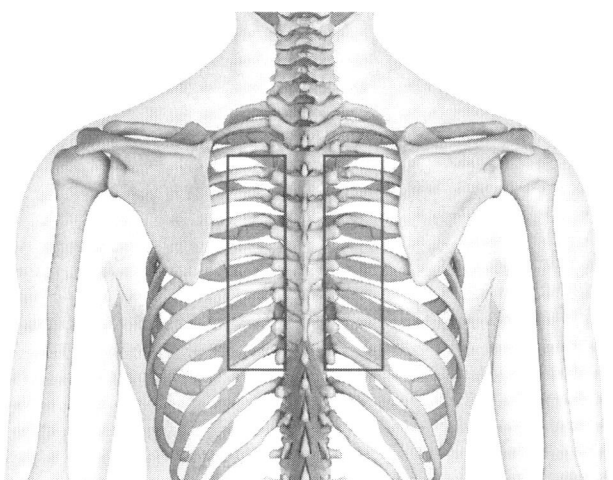

Fig. 7-6. DT.05

DT.06 Jiu Hou (Nine Monkeys) for scarlet fever

DT.06 is described as 18 points bilaterally. They include UB12, UB13, UB14, UB41, UB42, UB43, a point 3 cun lateral to T1, a point 6 cun lateral to T2, and a point 6 cun lateral to T3.

DT.06 is specifically for scarlet fever. I have no personal experience treating scarlet fever but as always, I would not take the precise points too literally. Rather, palpate in the general area of these points, and wet-cup the most tender point or points.

DT.07 San Jin (Three Metals) for knee problems

For painful knees, you will not find a more powerful or consistent treatment than bleeding the Master Tung "point" DT.07. It is surprisingly effective for advanced osteoarthritis of the knee, even when the patient has been told their knee is "bone on bone" and has failed all conventional therapies.

DT.07 is often described as a "3-point unit." The points are described as 3 cun lateral to the spine, in the 3rd, 4th, and 5th intercostal spaces.

In reality, it makes more sense to simply define DT.07 as an area, the "knee area." Palpate within that area to find the most tender spot, then bleed (wet-cup) there.

The area in which to palpate is pictured in Fig. 7-7 below. I've made it a little larger than the area typically described. Palpate within this area ipsilateral to the knee pain, bleed where it is most tender to palpation, and you cannot miss getting outstanding results.

If you simply cannot find a tender point in this area then it is not a blood stasis problem in this patient, and bleeding will not work. In that case, you will have to treat your patient with a different approach—possibly more local bleeding on the leg itself. That is all the more likely if you are dealing with a knee injury rather than a degenerative process.

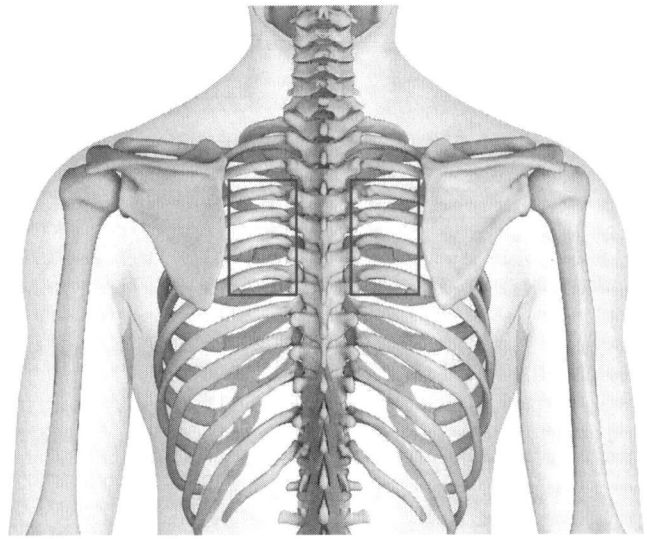

Fig. 7-7. DT.07 for pain in the knee, particularly from degenerative knee conditions.

DT.08 Jing Zhi (Essence Branch) and DT.09 Jin Lin (Metal Forest) for sciatica and lower limb problems

DT.08 is described as a "two point unit," 6 cun lateral to the spine, at the level of T2 and T3. It is for "Distention and pain in legs." DT.09 is described as 3 points, also 6 cun lateral to the spine, at the levels of the 4th, 5th and 6th intercostal spaces. It is for sciatica.

In practice, however, the points to be bled are found more medially, close to the medial border of the scapula. It makes more sense to amalgamate DT.08 and DT.09 into one area—as pictured in Fig. 7-8 below. Palpate within this area to find the most tender point in patients with leg pain and numbness.

As always when bleeding the back, if you palpate within this area and cannot find a tender point, then bleeding will not work for this patient.

Bleeding the back

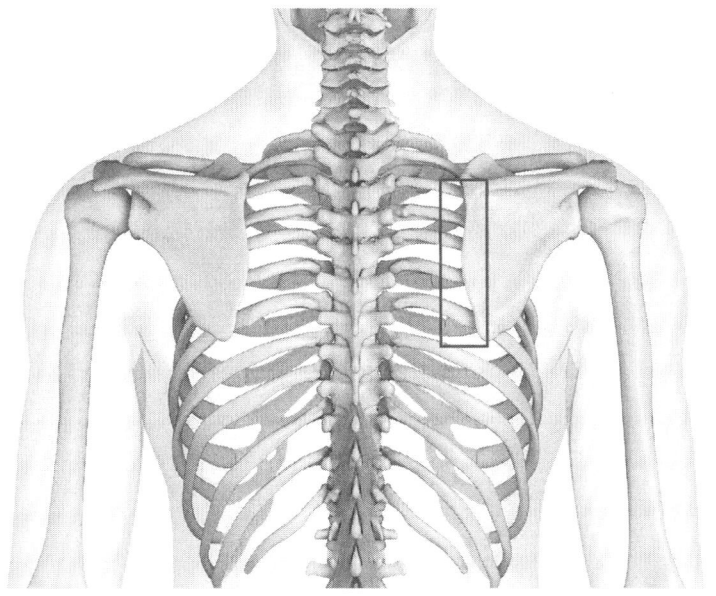

Fig. 7-8. DT.08-DT.09 for sciatica and pain in the lower extremities.

Upper limb zone for upper limb problems

The Master Tung point 44.17 (equivalent to the TCM point SI10) is an important point to bleed for problems of the ipsilateral upper limb.

However, I have often found points tender to palpation in that general area—not necessarily right at 44.17/SI10—on patients with upper limb issues. Bleeding those tender points wherever I find them in that area has been effective, particularly if the issue is any type of radiating pain or "nerve pain," but also a wide variety of problems typically diagnosed as "carpal tunnel syndrome." This includes pain, numbness and tingling in the hands, pain in the wrist, pain in the CMC joint, etc.

I am depicting this area as the "upper limb zone," shown in Fig. 7-9 below. Palpate within that area for upper limb problems, and wet-cup the most tender point. If you cannot find a point tender to palpation, bleeding in the area will not be effective.

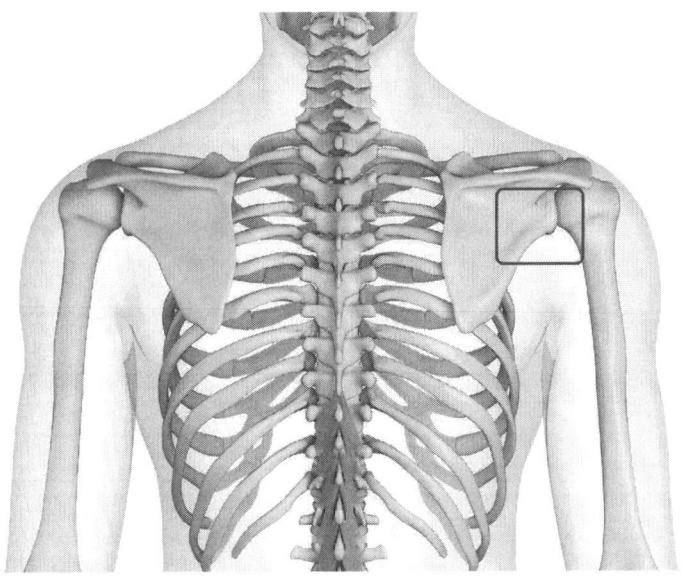

Fig. 7-9. Upper limb zone

Lung zone for respiratory problems

The area between the scapula and spine is wonderful to bleed for asthma, bronchitis, and other respiratory problems. Palpate that area, which includes DT.07 and the area just above and below it. I typically find 4 very tender points in patients with respiratory issues, two on each side, and wet-cup those. Patients usually get immediate relief in acute situations, and longer relief of chronic issues as well.

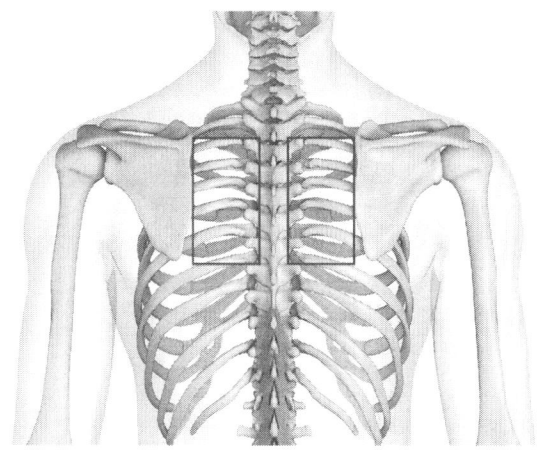

Fig. 7-10. Lung zone

Bleeding locally for upper back pain

Not infrequently, patients will present with a sharp, stabbing pain in the upper back. Typically the painful point is between the spine and scapula on the traps, but is sometimes on the scapula as well.

If the point is painful to palpation, the first thing I will do is dry-cup it. If that does not work, the next thing I do is wet-cup the painful point directly. More often than not, this will greatly ameliorate or resolve the problem.

Mid- and low back

DT.10 Ding Zhu (Top Pillar) for acute low back sprain and pain on breathing

DT.10 is described as two lines on each side of the mid-back, from T5 to T10, 3 cun lateral and 6 cun lateral. In reality, you can think of it as that whole area, as shown in Fig. 7-11 below.

Palpate this area, and bleed any very tender points you find. The area is bled for low back pain including acute back sprain, and pain in the chest when breathing.

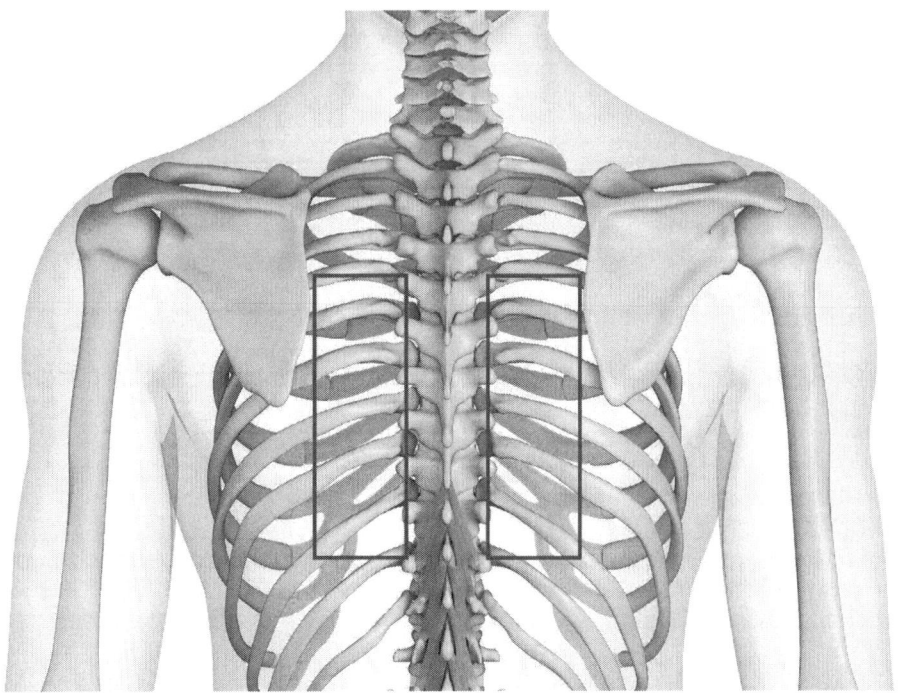

Fig. 7-11. DT.10 zone

DT.11 Hou Xin (Back of Heart)

DT.11 describes the area on the back from 3 cun to the left of the spine to 3 cun to the right of the spine, T5 to T10. Palpate that area and bleed (wet-cup) tender points for heart failure, gastric disorders, severe colds, acute eruptive diseases, abscesses, and finger numbness.

Bleeding the back

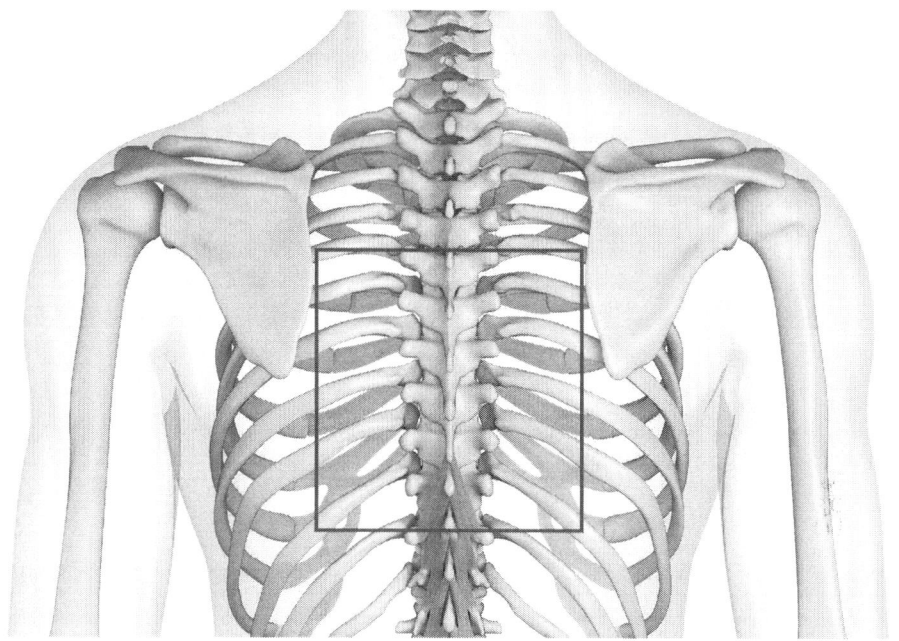

Fig. 7-12. DT.11 zone

DT.12 Gan Mao San (Common Cold) for severe colds

DT.12 is specifically for severe colds. Palpate for tender points in 3 areas—approximately 3 cun to the left and right of T4, and on the spine between T1 and T2, and wet-cup where tender.

The Complete Guide to Chinese Medicine Bloodletting

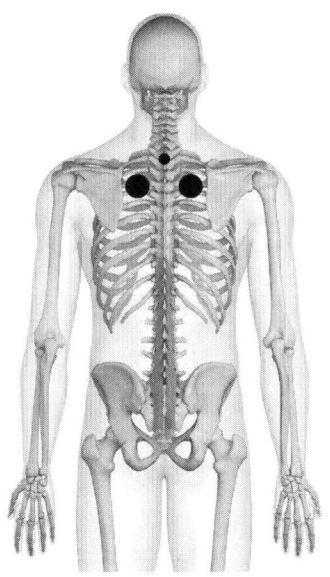

Fig. 7-13. DT.12

DT.13 Shui Zhong (Water Center) and DT.14 Shui Fu (Water Bowel) especially for kidney and reproductive issues (and more)

DT.13 and DT.14 are both for indications related to the kidneys and reproduction, and are best amalgamated into one zone.

Palpate approximately 1.5 cun lateral to the spine, from approximately L1 to L2. In addition to kidney disease and deficiency, this area can treat irregular menstruation and amenorrhea, constipation, impotence, headache, and bladder conditions.

Bleeding the back

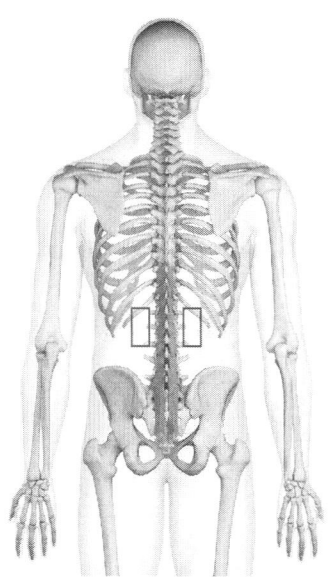

Fig. 7-14. DT13-14 zone

DT.15 San Jiang (Three Rivers) for gynecological issues and IBD

DT.15 is the large area from 3 cun to the right and left of the spine, and L2 to S3.

Palpate and bleed (wet-cup) tender points to treat food poisoning or acute flareup of IBD, also gynecological conditions such as amenorrhea, uterine inflammation and vaginal discharge.

The Complete Guide to Chinese Medicine Bloodletting

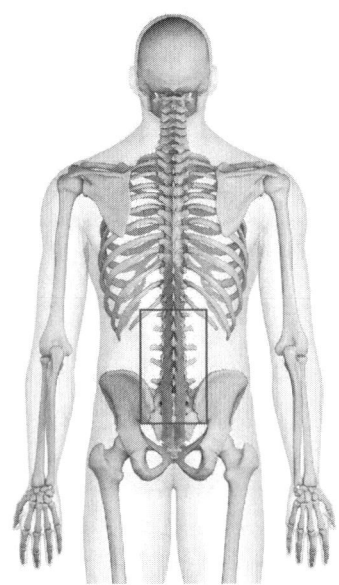

Fig. 7-15. DT.15 zone

DT.16 Shuang He (Dual Rivers) for upper limb issues

DT.16 describes two lines on the low back—each 3 cun lateral to the spine, from L2 to S3. Palpate along those lines and bleed (wet-cup) any very tender points for pain of the upper limbs and shoulder.

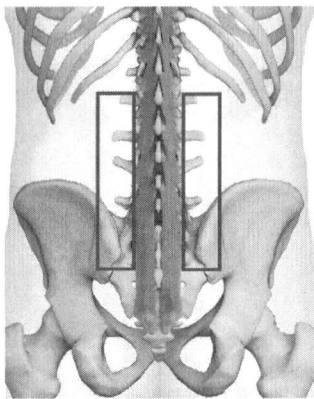

Fig. 7-16. DT.16 zone

DT.17 Chong Xiao (Rushing to Heaven) for occipital headaches

DT.17 comprises the line on the DU channel from S3 to the coccyx. This is specifically for pain in the back of the head; i.e. occipital headaches. Palpate and bleed (wet-cup) any tender points you find.

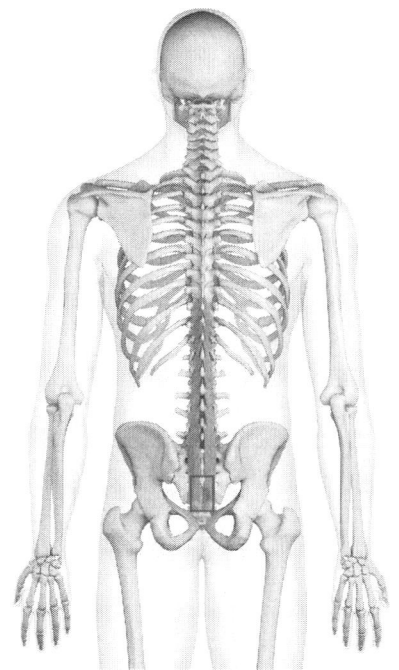

Fig. 7-17. DT.17 zone

UB 18 for nosebleeds

UB18 is at the level of T9, 1.5 cun lateral to the spine. Bleeding that point is specific for nosebleeds. I have not had to bleed that point often but when I have, it has been amazingly effective.

Palpate in that area until you find the point, which will be very tender to palpation, and wet-cup ipsilateral to the side where the nosebleed is occurring or—in the case of chronic recurring nosebleeds—the side where it keeps occurring. Bleed bilaterally for nosebleeds in both nostrils.

UB 20 and UB 21 for rosacea

UB20 is at the level of T11 and UB21 is at the level of T12, 1.5 cun lateral to the spine. Bleeding there is specific for rosacea.

Palpate in that area until you find a point on each side very tender to palpation, and bleed (wet-cup).

Supplies/tools for bleeding the back

Safety lancets

Prior to the use of safety lancets, wet-cupping was far more challenging for both patients and practitioners. Acupuncturists used 3-edge needles, and had to prepare patients for the pain they would experience. Often they were told to cough at the moment of puncture to minimize the pain.

The use of safety lancets has changed that. The needles are so sharp and the spring action so quick that patients feel nothing. In my experience they do not even know they've been lanced unless you tell them.

Safety lancets also have the wonderful property of being absolutely safe for your patients and for you. They can only be activated one time, so cross-contamination by accidental needlestick is impossible.

The largest-diameter safety lancets are the 17 gauge lancets, and these are the ones I use and highly recommend. There are two manufacturers of this size lancet. The yellow and white ones pictured in Chapter 2 are sold under the name McKesson in North America, and Acti-Lance elsewhere in the world.

Another brand of 17g safety lancet I have found equally effective is the Capiject brand, made by Terumo.

If you cannot obtain these lancets, you can use a higher gauge than 17g (the higher the gauge, the smaller the diameter of the needle), but you will have to use a more of them. It is not quite the same however—best is to use the larger size.

Cups

You can use glass fire cups, or you can use plastic pump cups. I find it faster and easier to use plastic cups.

If you use glass cups you need to sterilize them after each use, which is time-consuming. You can save time by using inexpensive single-use disposable plastic cups.

In the US, you can buy DongBang sterile disposable cups for $0.25 each. Use once and discard. Besides saving time, the use of single-use disposable cups is the highest standard of safety for your patients.

If you are not in the US, you can buy them at a good price through Alibaba.com from Worldtech Co. Ltd. See Appendix I—Supplies for more details. This company can sell you the DongBang cups and pumps that fit them. I have ordered from them and found them to be reliable, but I have no relationship with them.

As noted earlier, one can buy plastic inserts as pictured in Fig. 7-18 below, but you should not use them for wet-cupping. The extra layer of plastic between the cup and the skin makes the vacuum seal unreliable, and air can leak into the cup. When it does, suction will be lost and you will end up with a bloody mess.

Also, you are handling the cup with gloves that will sometimes have blood on them so you still end up with blood on the outside of the cup, meaning you have to sterilize it, and no good way of doing so.

If you use a plastic cup for bloodletting, best is to just throw it out when you are done.

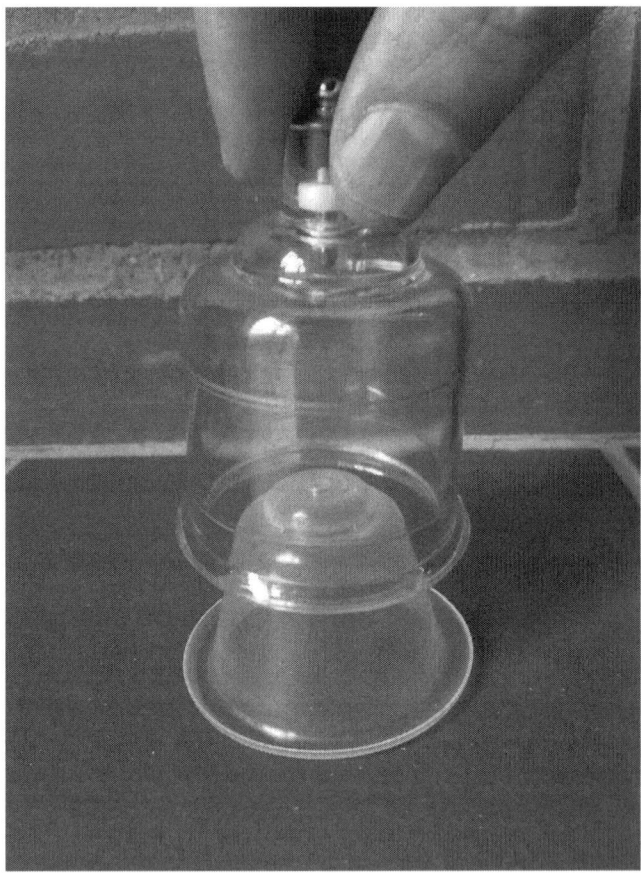

Fig. 7-18. For several reasons, the use of these cup inserts for bloodletting is not recommended.

Plastic bags to protect your pump

Assuming you're using single-use disposable cups and single-use disposable safety lancets, wet-cupping is extremely safe, with almost no chance of cross-infection of blood-borne disease.

But there's still one "weak link" in the chain of possible cross-infection that we haven't discussed. The potential problem is the pump.

Why the pump? Because during the wet-cupping procedure, you will sometimes get blood on your gloves, and you will touch the pump. If your patient is positive for hepatitis B—which is EXTREMELY infectious—some viable viruses will get on the pump. You will then touch that pump the next time you wet-cup,

Bleeding the back

and you could get the previous patient's viruses on your new set of gloves, and touch your new patient with them—possibly right where you're about to lance.

There is an easy fix that can solve that weak link, and make your wet-cupping process virtually perfect. Just place the pump in a plastic bag before you start, and handle it only through the bag. Then discard the bag when you are done.

In my bleeding room I have a roll of plastic bags hanging on a paper towel rack, as pictured in Fig. 7-19. The roll fits on the towel rack perfectly. See Appendix I—Supplies for more information.

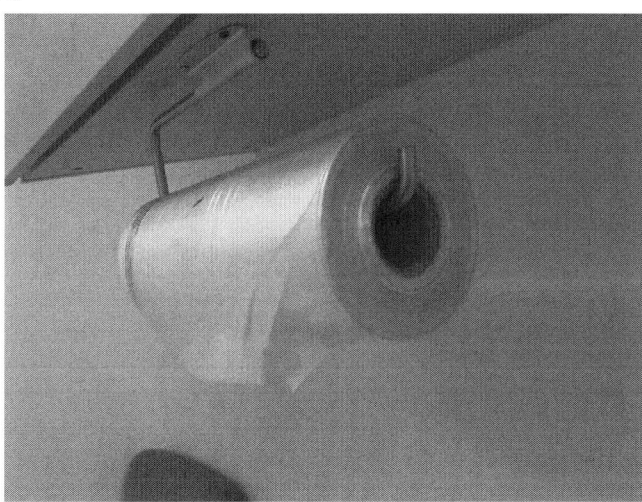

Fig. 7-19.

The Complete Guide to Chinese Medicine Bloodletting

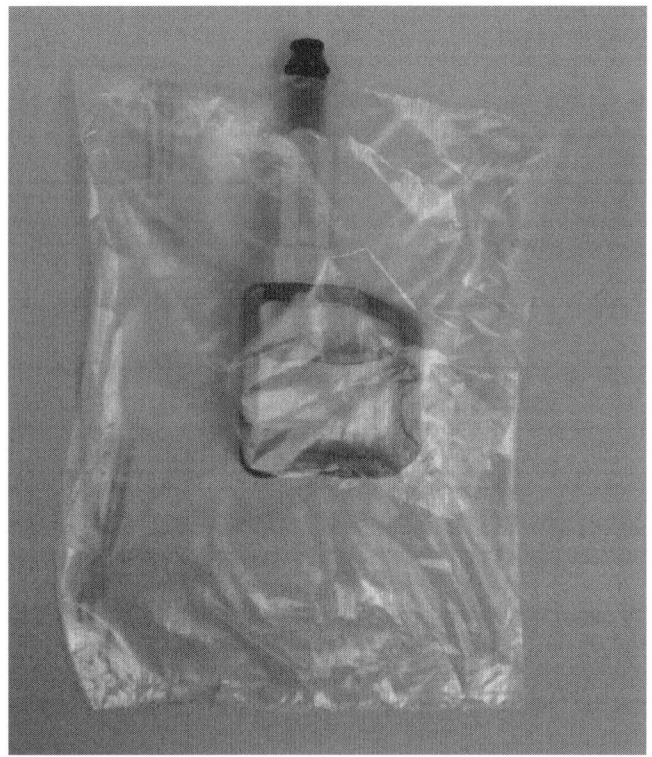

Fig. 7-20.

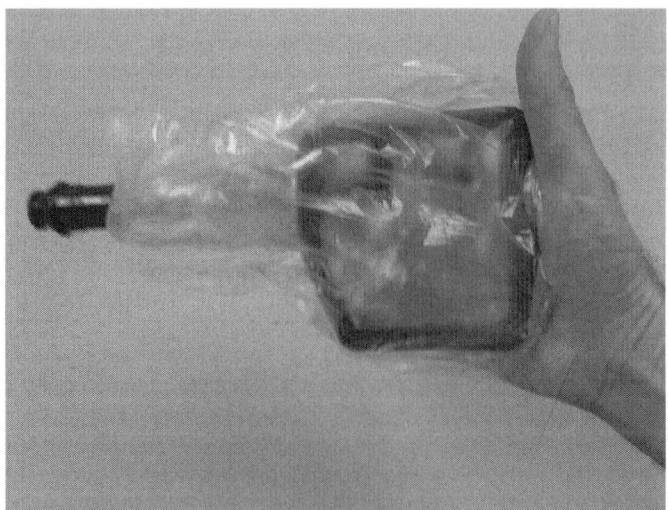

Fig. 7-21.

Step-by-step instructions for bleeding the back

Prepare your clean field with 4-5 safety lancets, a few cotton balls or gauze (clean or sterile), clean cup, pump for cup inside of plastic bag, bandages, and packaged alcohol wipes.

Put on gloves. Clean the area you are about to "let" with an alcohol wipe. Take a safety lancet and twist the plastic stopper ¼ turn to remove and ready for use.

With your thumb, palpate the patient's back to find the MOST TENDER point. Keep palpating until you are certain you have found it. If the patient says "Yeah, around there"—that's not good enough. Keep palpating until the patient flinches and says "There!" with certainty. Anything less is not good enough—take your time and find the very best spot.

Place your safety lancet on that exact spot, press the button, and discard. Palpate around that spot again until you find a tender spot, and continue until you've used all 4 or 5 lancets. Keep in mind that the punctures should be sufficiently close together that they can all fit within the 2" diameter of the cup.

This should be done fairly quickly. If it takes more than 15 seconds or so from the first puncture to the time the cup goes on, the blood may start to clot. A quick swipe with an alcohol swab will remove any clot that is forming, thin the blood a bit, and help blood flow.

Place the cup over the punctures and pump out air. The amount of blood you get will vary widely from patient to patient. You should get enough blood that some runs down and gathers at the inside rim of the cup. If that doesn't happen, you can remove the cup and swab the puncture area with alcohol, which thins the blood and encourages flow.

When you have enough blood, remove the cup carefully to avoid spillage. Discard the blood according to local regulations, along with any blood-tinged paper towels and cotton. Remove the pump from the plastic bag, and discard the bag.

I generally do not leave cups on for more than 5 minutes or so, and sometimes less. However much blood you get during that time is sufficient.

Removing wet cups from the back without spilling blood

Following are detailed instructions for removing the cup without spilling blood.

People's backs are curved, so generally the cup is not really flat on the back, it's at an angle, and blood gathers at the low edge.

Roll two or three sheets of paper towel into a "rope," wrap that rope around the lower edge, and use that as a fulcrum or hinge.

The lower edge of the cup will stay in contact with the skin, again, acting as a "hinge." As you lift off the upper edge, the blood will flow into the cup. Once it does, you can remove it.

Try not to turn the cup all the way upside down because if it flows into the valve, it can leak out.

If you sop up the blood in sufficient paper towels or cotton that you cannot squeeze out a drop, then you can double-bag it and throw it out with normal trash (if local regulations permit).

If the cup is truly flat on the patient's back, you can have the patient turn a little so their back is at an angle. Another technique is to release the suction and slide the cup to a more slanted area on the patient's back, being careful to keep the edges of the cup in contact with the patient's skin so as not to let blood leak out of the cup. The motion is the same as that used when slide-cupping

When you are done, discard the plastic cup. Having come into contact with blood, it cannot be adequately sterilized and should not be reused.

Bleeding the back

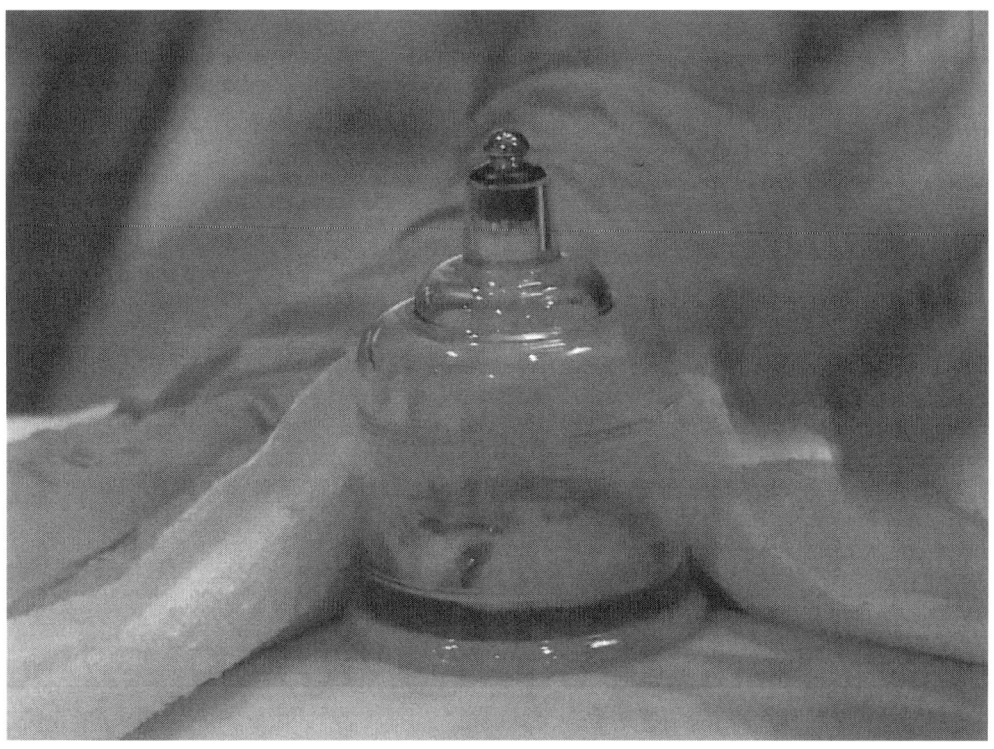

Fig. 7-22. Place rolled up paper towels around the lower edge of the cup. *Full-color picture at www.chinesebloodletting.com.*

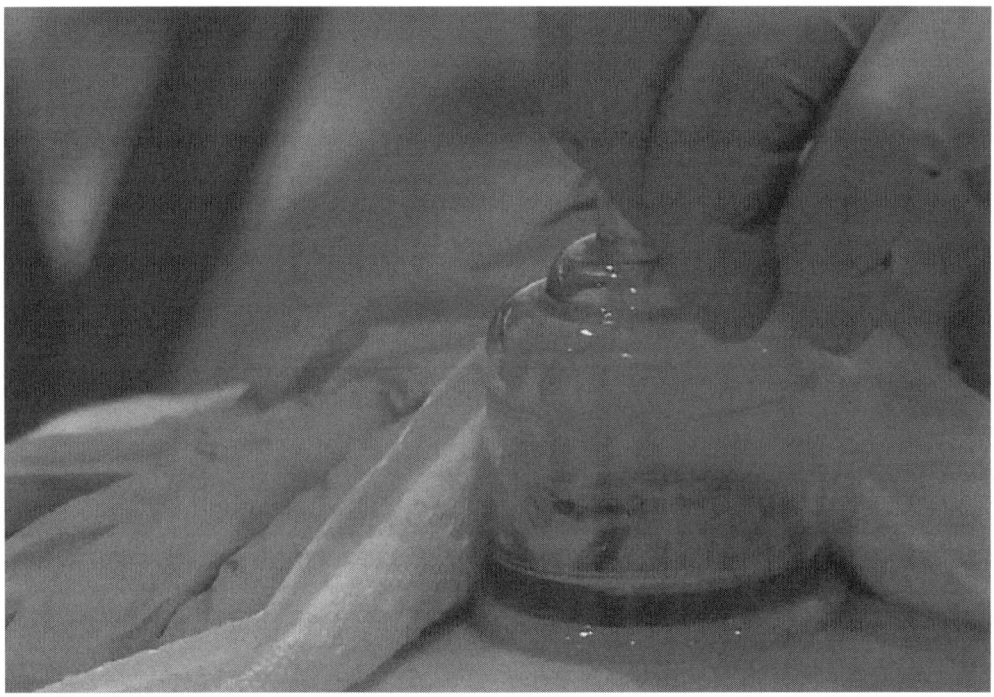

Fig. 7-23. If using a plastic cup, pull up the valve at the top of the cup to release suction. *Full-color picture at www.chinesebloodletting.com.*

Bleeding the back

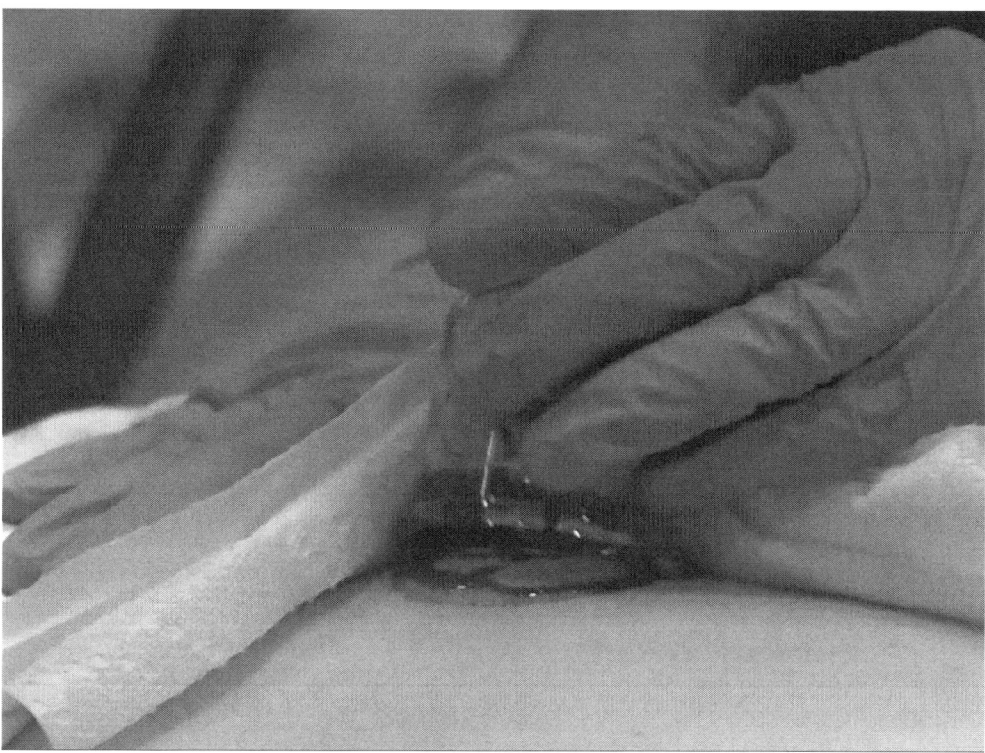

Fig. 7-24. Press down gently on the skin with the lower lip of the cup and carefully tilt the cup toward the lower edge. *Full-color picture at www.chinesebloodletting.com.*

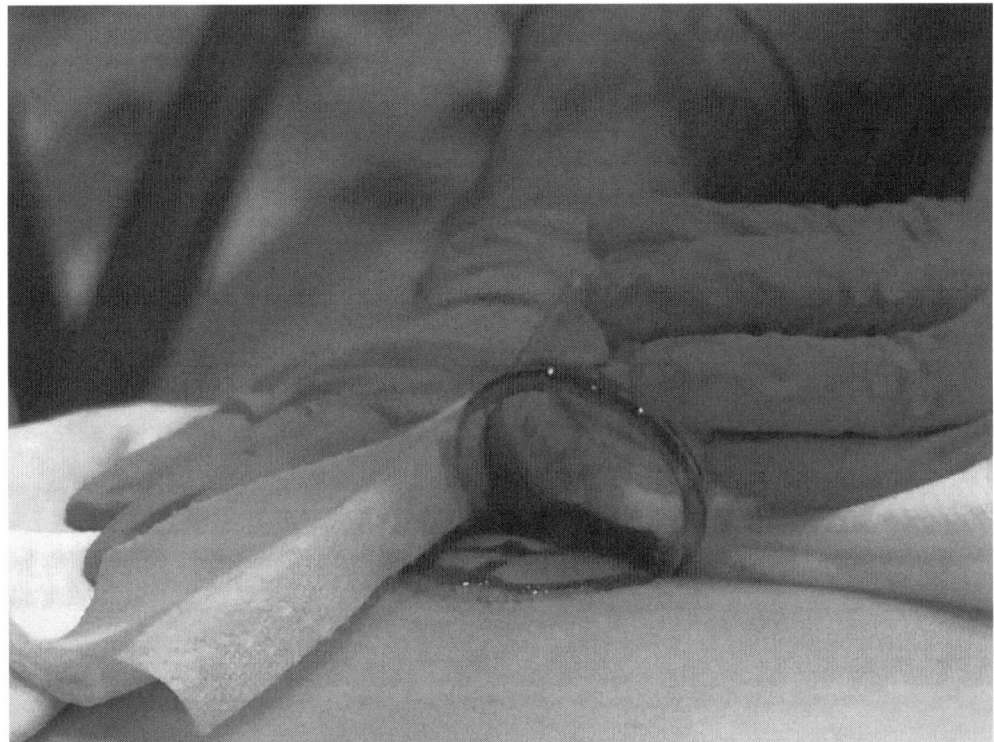

Fig. 7-25. *Full-color picture at www.chinesebloodletting.com.*

Bleeding the back

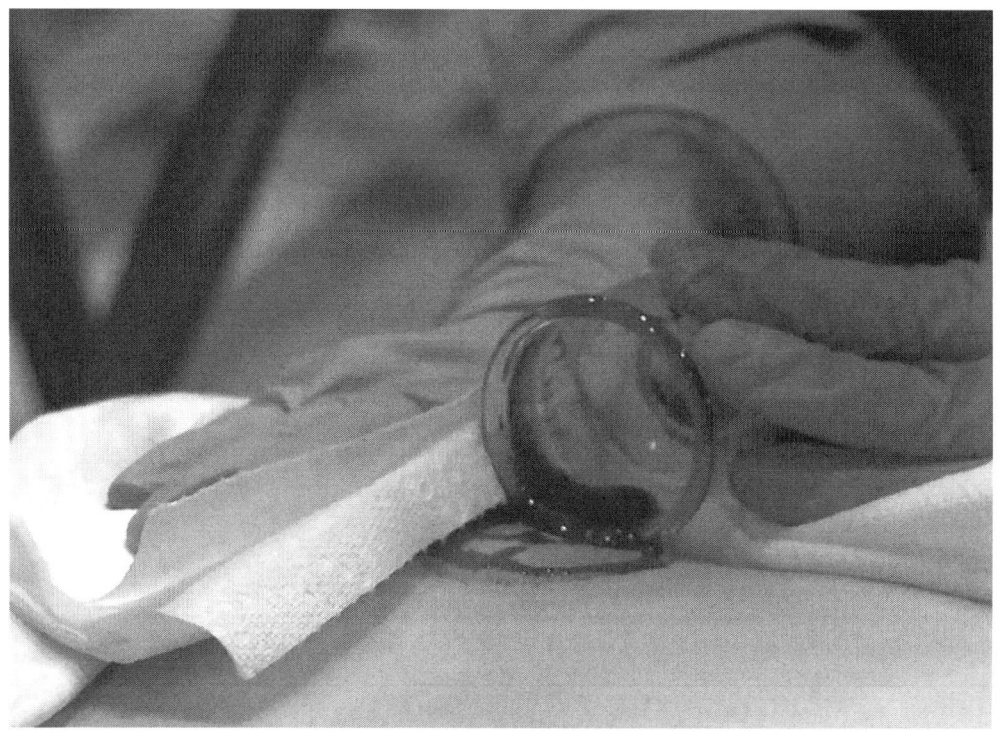

Fig. 7-26. *Full-color picture at www.chinesebloodletting.com.*

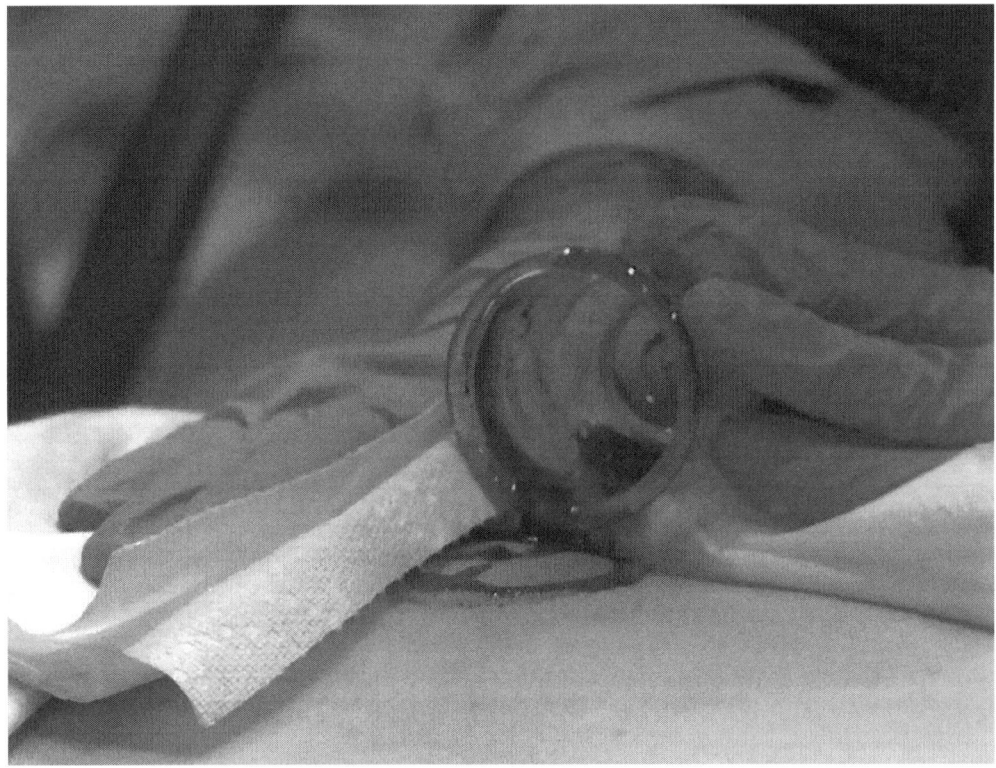

Fig. 7-27. Once the contents are in the cup, you can remove it, place a wad of paper towels or cotton into the cup to soak up the blood, and discard. *Full-color picture at www.chinesebloodletting.com.*

When can I bleed the back again?

Let's imagine your patient comes in complaining of right knee pain. You palpate their right DT.07 area, find a very tender spot, bleed (wet-cup) it, and the patient feels better, but still not 100%.

What is your plan now? When can you have the patient come back for more bleeding and further relief?

The answer is—pretty soon, even a few days later. While you don't want to bleed the same spot more than once every 3 weeks or so, the interesting thing about bleeding the back is this: the next time your patient comes in, palpate in a circle around the area where you bled the last time (the puncture marks should still be visible) and you will find a new "most tender" spot. Bleed that.

Bleeding the back

I don't know by what magic a new tender spot always develops near the previous one, but it never fails. That new tender spot is apparently another aspect of the blood stasis that caused the problem in the first place, and you can further treat and remove that blood stasis by bleeding the new tender point.

Here are two pictures that illustrate this. Fig. 7-28 shows the DT.07 area on the back of a patient who came in for knee pain a week earlier. At that initial appointment I bled DT.07 and he left with no pain. When he came back a week later, that knee had begun acting up again.

You can see the faint cup mark from the previous appointment and the faint puncture marks. I palpated all around those, and found a very tender point which I punctured. This picture was taken just after the punctures and before cupping. This was several weeks ago and he has had no knee pain since, although he has come in for other issues.

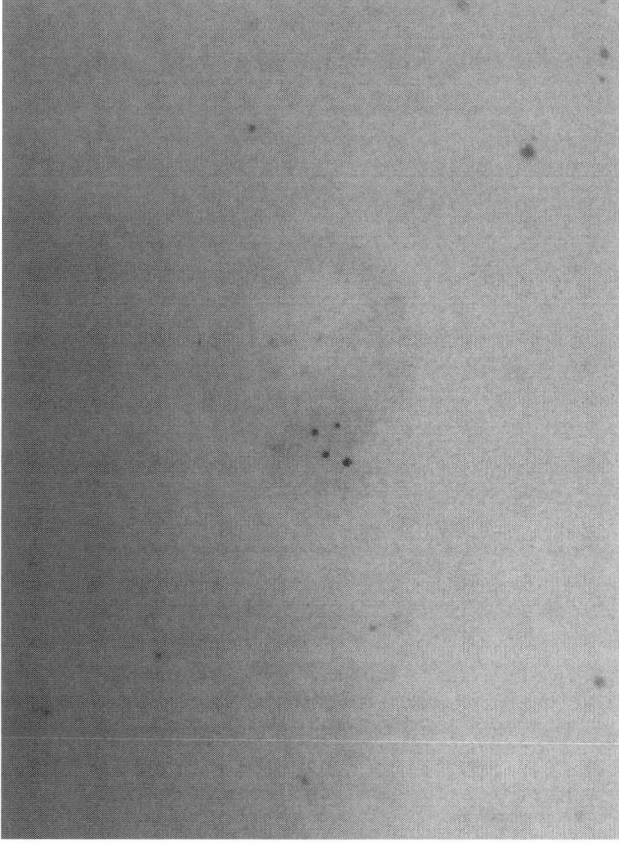

Fig. 7-28. *Full-color picture at www.chinesebloodletting.com.*

Fig. 7-29 shows the back of a woman who comes in for sciatica. You can see the dark cupping mark and punctures from 5 days earlier, and also where I found a new tender point and cupped.

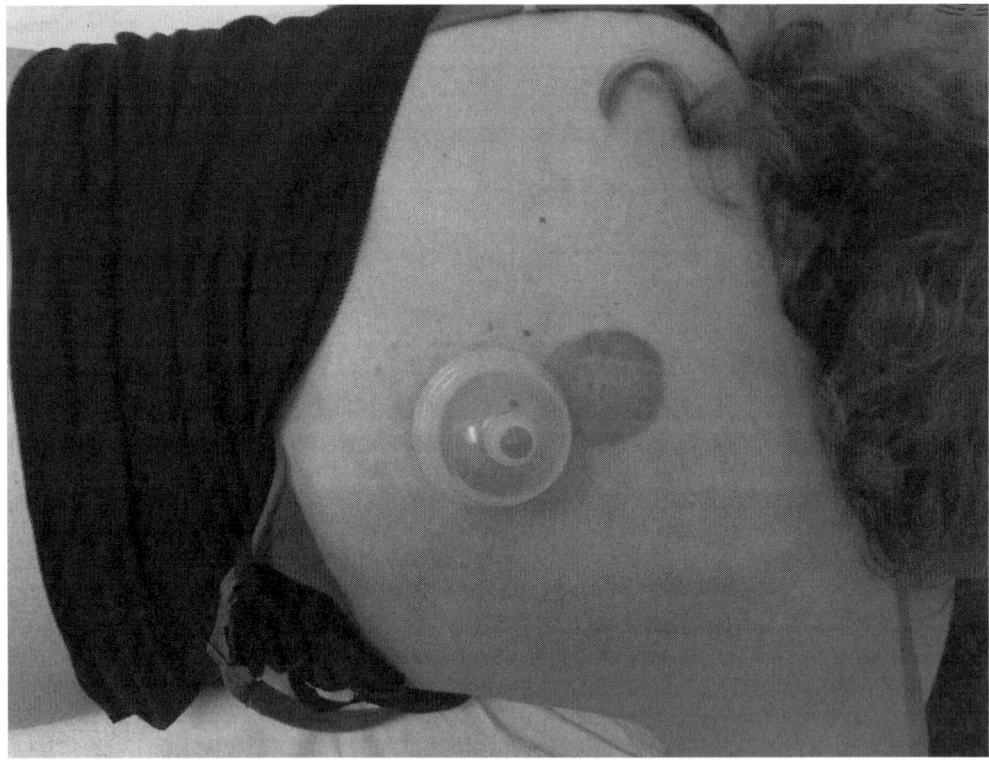

Fig. 7-29. The dark cupping mark is from 5 days earlier. *Full-color picture at www.chinesebloodletting.com.*

Predicting the efficacy of bleeding the back

Before bleeding

Palpating for tender points tells you whether or not to bleed the back, where to bleed the back, and how likely it is that bleeding the back will be effective.

Again, if you palpate the back and find no tender points, there is no reason to bleed. It will not be effective.

Assuming you do find a point tender to palpation in the appropriate area, however, the effectiveness of bleeding will be directly proportional to how tender that point is. If the patient "jumps off the table" when you palpate that point—especially if the mirror-image point on the contralateral side is not tender at all—you are virtually guaranteed success.

During bleeding

On some patients, your cup will fill with blood fairly quickly. On others, you will barely get a drop.

Generally speaking, a good flow of blood is associated with a positive response. This is not a hard-and-fast rule however. It can also happen that patients with minimal blood flow respond favorably. Tenderness to palpation is a more reliable guide.

Chapter 8

Bleeding legs

Unlike the back, most people's legs have visible veins. They may be obvious and dark—like purple spider veins—or they may be greenish and faint.

Either way, when you bleed legs, you are bleeding veins. Use a bleeding needle (preferably a hypodermic needle) to directly prick a vein and let it bleed.

As we learned in Chapter 7 however—with rare exceptions—there are no visible veins on the back.

That difference—visible veins on the legs vs no visible veins on the back—is why bleeding legs is very different from bleeding the back.

When you bleed legs—since you are bleeding visible veins—your EYES are your guide. You use your eyes to determine the exact point to prick. You are looking for the most obvious, darkest veins.

Ideal veins to bleed are dark purple spider veins, as in the picture below. Unlike when you bleed the back, you do not use palpation to find points to bleed on the legs.

Fig. 8-1 below shows "ideal" veins to bleed. Such veins are good to bleed because they are clear signs of blood stasis and thus bleeding them is likely to benefit your patient. The blood that comes out is dark, another sign of probable success. These veins are very superficial and thus easy to bleed. Since they are just below the surface, blood has a short distance to travel before exiting the body, meaning little chance to extravasate into surrounding tissue, i.e. little or no bruising.

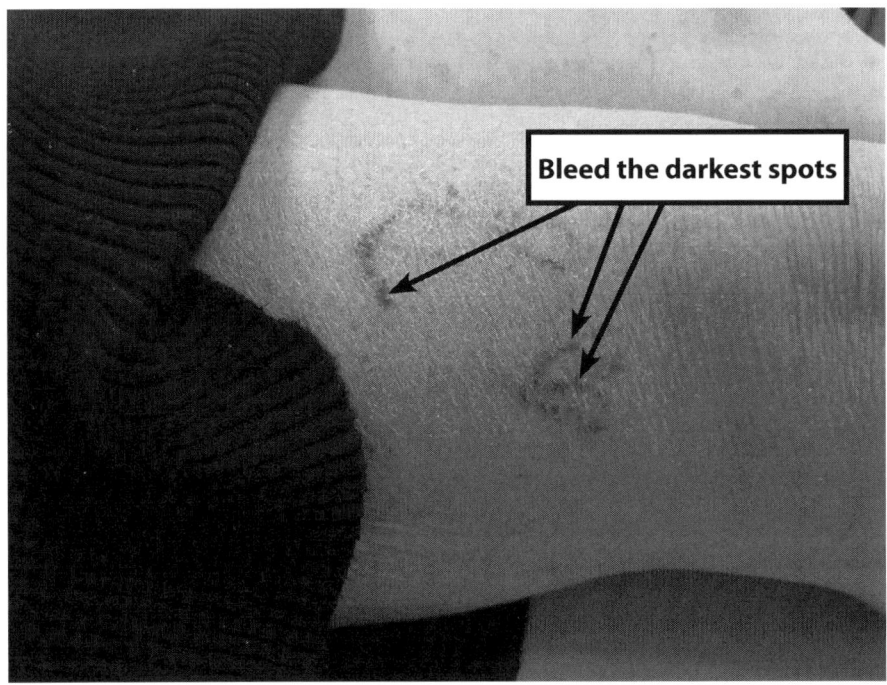

Fig. 8-1. "Ideal" veins for bleeding. You could bleed any points along these veins; the arrows point to a few good choices. *Full-color picture at www.chinesebloodletting.com.*

Sometimes there are no "perfect" veins on a patient's leg—in that case you have to find the most visible vein you can. But always when bleeding legs you are looking for—and pricking—veins.

Since you are bleeding veins and have to be precise, you cannot use a spring-loaded safety lancet. They are simply not precise enough, and you cannot aim with the exactness required. Moreover, it probably will not go deep enough.

For bleeding legs—which means bleeding veins—you have to use a manual device. I use—and highly recommend—18 gauge or 20 gauge hypodermic needles.

Since you are bleeding a vein directly, the blood will flow on its own. There is no need to cup.

So to sum up—when bleeding legs you are bleeding visible veins, your eyes are your final guide as to exactly where to prick, you use a manual instrument such as a hypodermic needle, and cupping is unnecessary.

CAUTION—Bleed veins that are flat, not veins that bulge!

Generally speaking you can safely bleed almost any visible vein in the legs. The exception is veins that bulge or protrude.

You particularly want to avoid bleeding ropey, knotty varicose veins such as those pictured in Figs. 8-2, 8-3, and 8.4 below. These are diseased veins whose valves are no longer functioning properly. If you bleed them you will get plenty of blood—more than you want—but bleeding them will produce no therapeutic effect and, in fact, will just make the veins even more swollen.

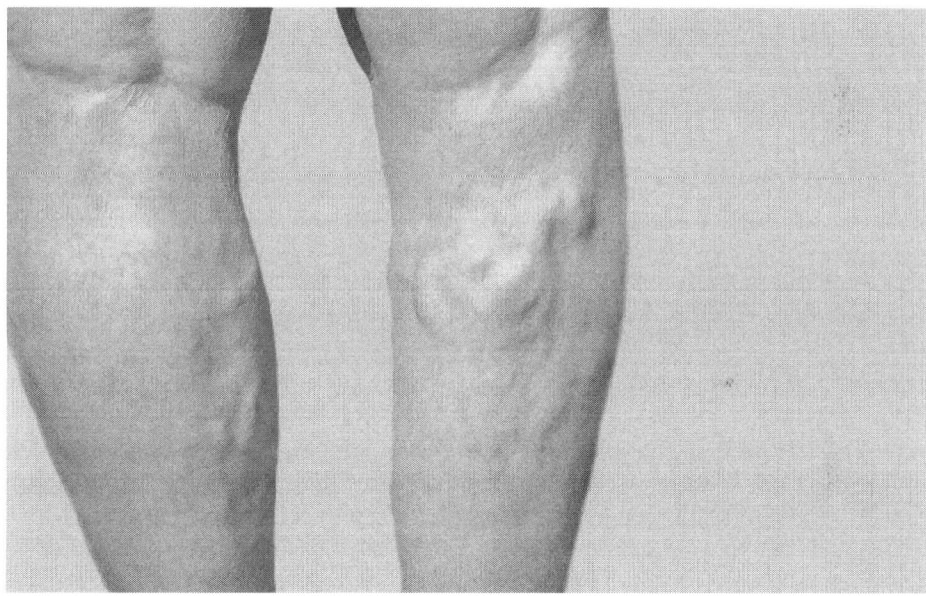

Fig. 8-2. *Full-color picture at www.chinesebloodletting.com.*

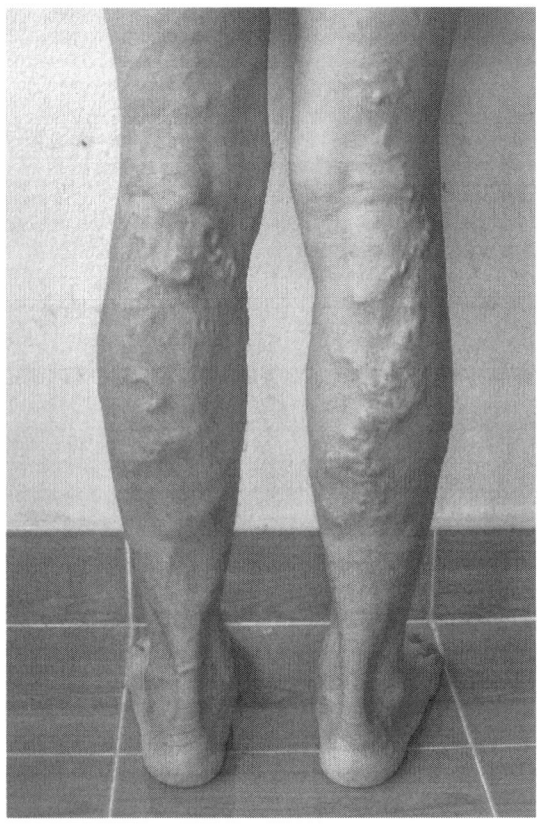

Fig. 8-3. Never directly bleed ropey, bulging varicose veins such as those in the above 2 pictures. *Full-color picture at www.chinesebloodletting.com.*

Bleeding legs

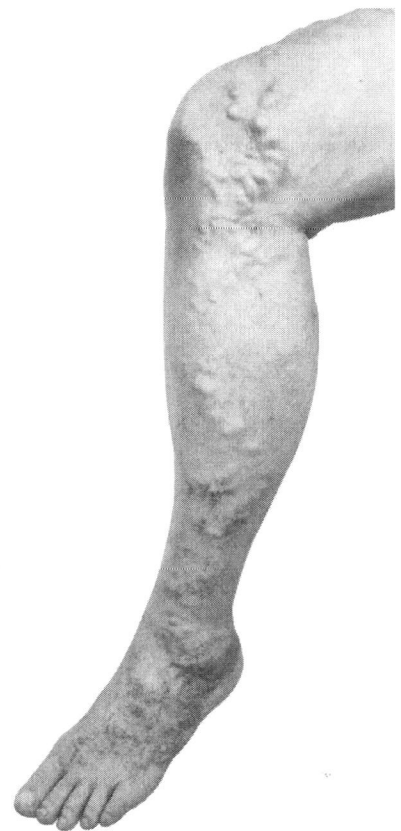

Fig. 8-4. Avoid bleeding ropey, bulging varicose veins such as those near the knee in the picture above. However, you can treat those varicose veins effectively by bleeding the dark, flat veins in the lower leg and foot. *Full-color picture at www.chinesebloodletting.com.*

The veins pictured in Fig. 8-5 below are not varicose veins but they protrude, so it is better to avoid them. Again, such veins have a tendency to swell and bruise.

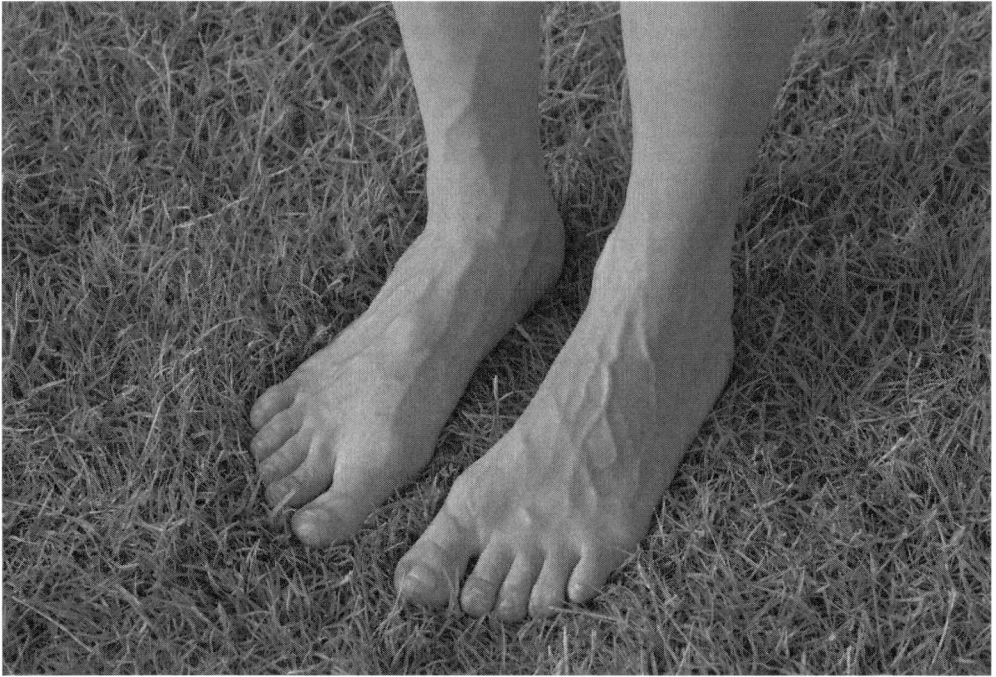

Fig. 8-5. *Full-color picture at www.chinesebloodletting.com.*

List of indications for bleeding legs

The legs are the most important and effective part of the body for bleeding. Symptoms in almost every part of the body can be effectively treated by bleeding veins in legs.

It is easier to list the indications for which you do not bleed legs than the ones for which you do.

One common problem for which I rarely bleed legs is knee pain, especially knee pain of degenerative origin. For that, the upper back DT.07 area is the go-to area to bleed. I can cite several examples of knee pain that did not respond to bleeding on the leg, but did respond spectacularly to bleeding DT.07.

Even for knees, however, on rare occasions I have better success bleeding the leg than bleeding DT.07. These patients tend to have atypical knee pain, where the pain, stiffness or swelling is "around" the knee rather than in the knee joint itself. The tendency is that DT.07 is for pain of a degenerative nature as in osteoarthritis, while for knee pain due to athletic injury you may have to bleed around the knee itself.

As always, let your eyes be your guide; bleed any dark, prominent veins you find on that leg and palpate the DT.07 area to see if you can find a very tender point.

For eye problems such as styes, ptosis, and optic neuritis, the go-to place to bleed is the apex of the ear. I generally don't bleed the leg for eye problems.

For almost every other issue that can be resolved with bloodletting, bleeding the legs can make a world of difference—particularly if the patient has obvious signs of blood stasis in their legs. In other words, if they have dark, prominent veins or—for that matter—any visible, flat (not bulging) veins.

Where to bleed legs

Earlier, I pointed out ways in which bleeding legs is different from bleeding the back.

One additional important difference is this; when bleeding the back, the areas to bleed for each indication are well-defined. For example, if a patient comes in with knee pain, the area to bleed is ALWAYS the DT.07 area on the upper back. It is NEVER the mid back or low back. It is NEVER in the middle of the scapula.

When bleeding legs,Tha however, it is not so clear which area should be bled for a particular problem. Rather, when bleeding legs, the ultimate answer to the question "Where should I bleed?" is "Bleed what you see." You should always bleed the darkest, most prominent veins you find, wherever on the leg you happen to find them.

In other words, when bleeding legs, FORGET ABOUT POINTS!!! Bleeding legs is NOT a matter of, for example, "bleed ST36." It is rather a matter of "look for visible veins in the general vicinity of ST36 and bleed if any are there." Or simply "Examine the patient's legs and bleed the most visible, darkest veins you find."

There are also Master Tung bleeding zones on the legs that can help guide you, as described in the next section. For example, the Master Tung stomach region (see page 121) is on the anterior ankle, in the area surrounding ST41.

In general, the most common place to bleed on the legs is behind the knee in the area surrounding UB40, the so-called Master Tung occipital zone. Perhaps the next most common place to bleed is the lateral leg, the area between the stomach channel and the GB channel.

In other words, the Tung bleeding zones provide you with an idea of where you might find the best veins to bleed for a particular condition. But always remember that the map is not the territory. Those bleeding zones are helpful but in the final analysis, "Bleed what you see." Bleed the darkest, most prominent veins you find—even if they're not where they're "supposed" to be.

Tung's bleeding zones and the conditions they treat

Following are diagrams of the Master Tung bleeding zones, or regions, of the leg. Remember that these are suggestive and not absolute. In the final analysis, when bleeding veins in the legs, the most important rule is "Bleed what you see."

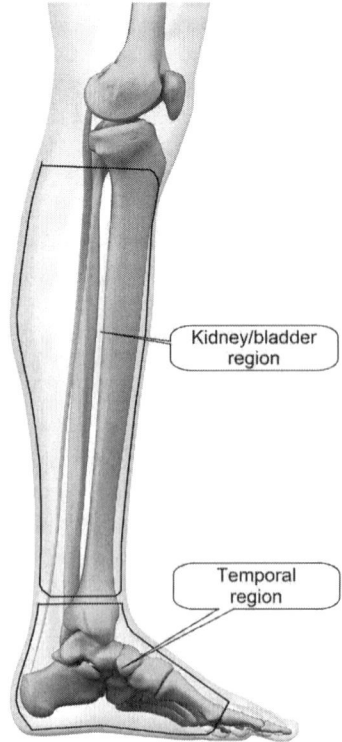

Fig. 8-6. Master Tung bleeding regions of the medial leg

Bleeding legs

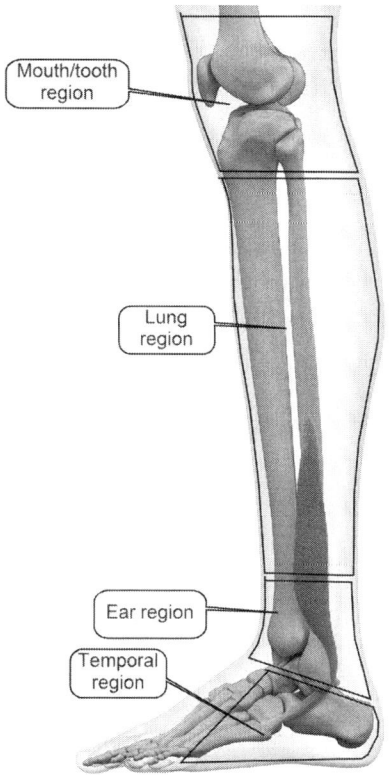

Fig. 8-7. Master Tung bleeding regions of the lateral leg

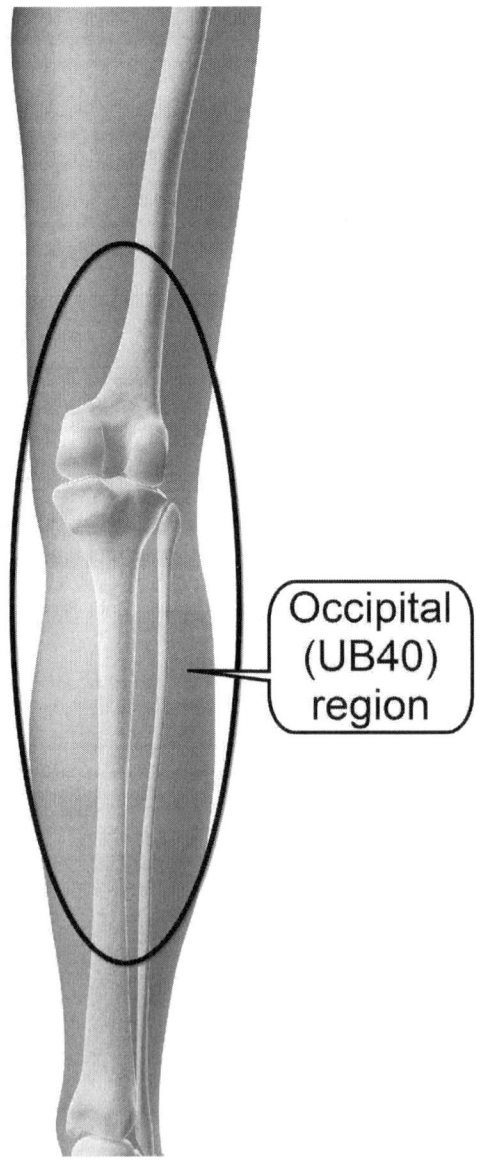

Fig. 8-8. Master Tung bleeding region of the posterior leg

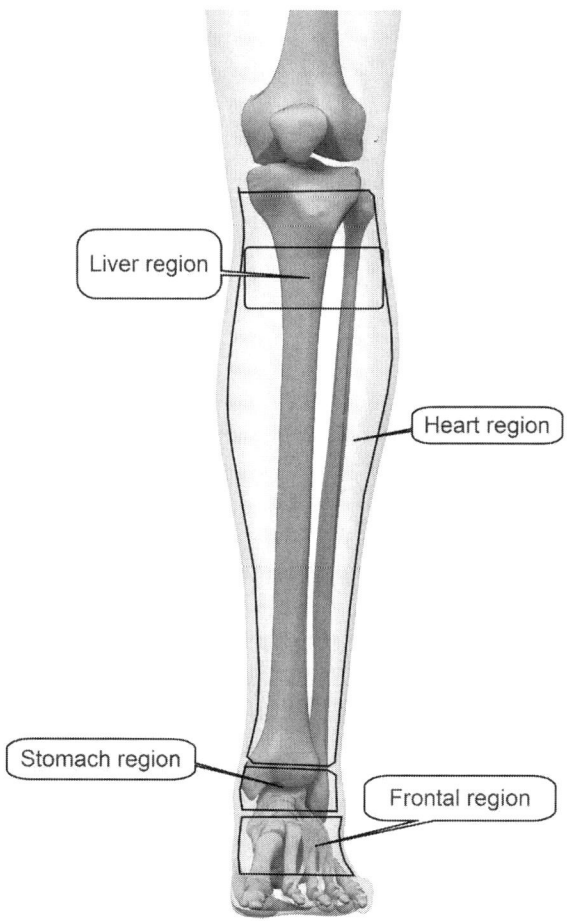

Fig. 8-9. Master Tung bleeding regions of the anterior leg

Veins to bleed and veins to avoid

Following is a gallery of veins, with commentary on how to bleed and whether to bleed.

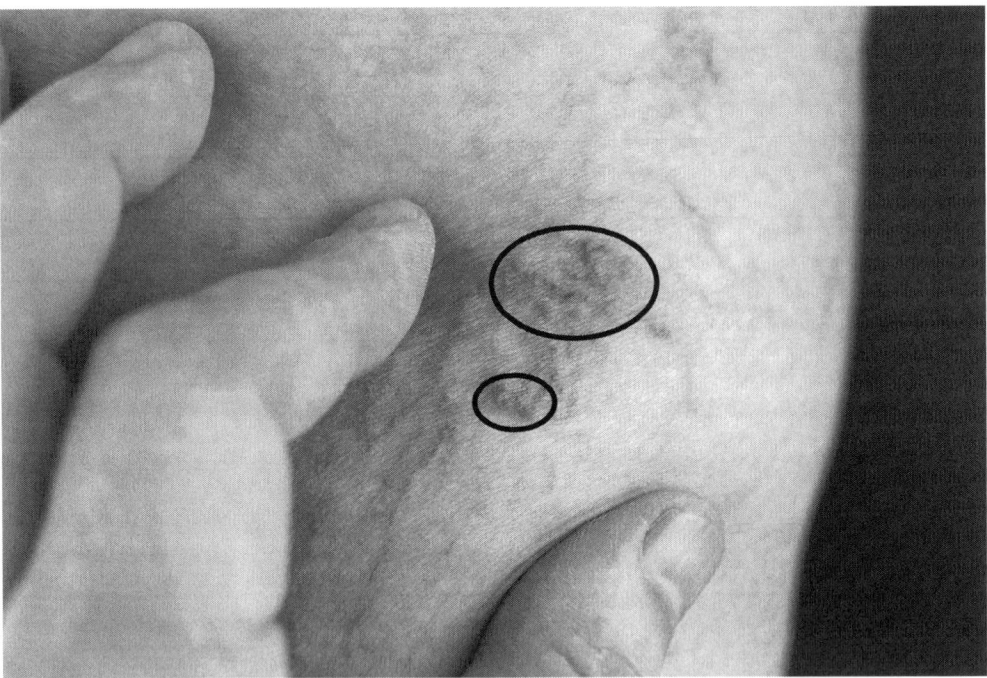

Fig. 8-10. These veins protrude a bit but they are not varicose veins, just a cluster of blood stasis, and they SHOULD be bled. Dark blood can ooze from such veins for a while so keep squeezing and wipe every 30 seconds or so with an alcohol swab to prevent a clot from forming, and keep the blood flowing until it's mostly done. Prick a dark spot in the lower circle first, then one or two in the upper circle—do not prick the upper circle first because the blood will make it hard to see the veins in the lower circle. *Full-color picture at www.chinesebloodletting.com.*

Bleeding legs

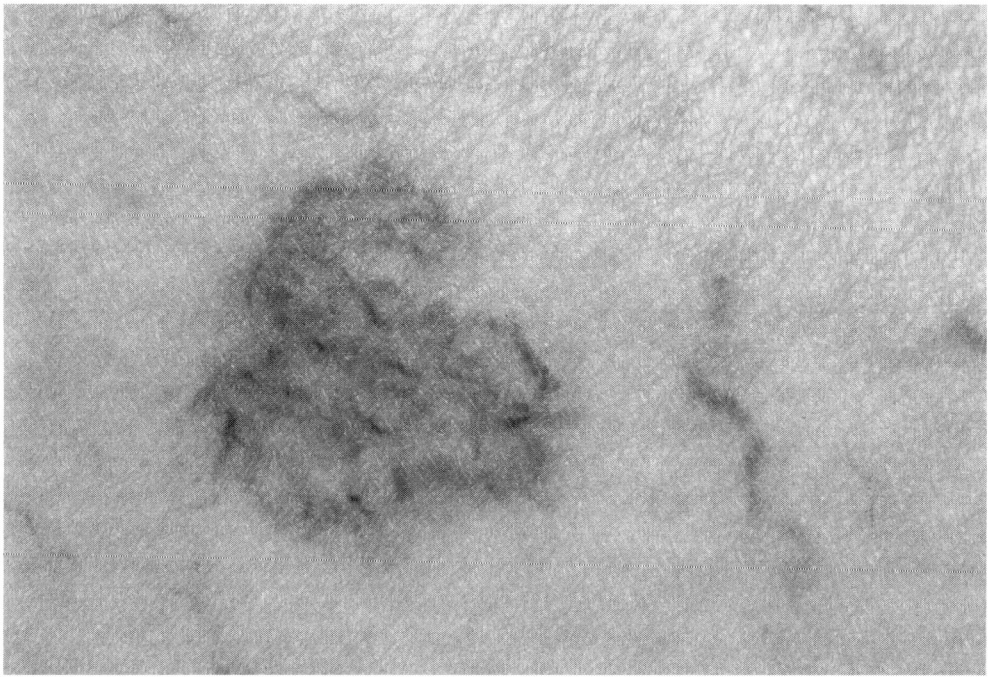

Fig. 8-11. This is a nice cluster of blood stasis that should be bled. Two or three pricks should suffice; be sure to bleed the lower points first so that flowing blood does not obscure your view. Superficial, dark veins such as these generally do not bruise. *Full-color picture at www.chinesebloodletting.com.*

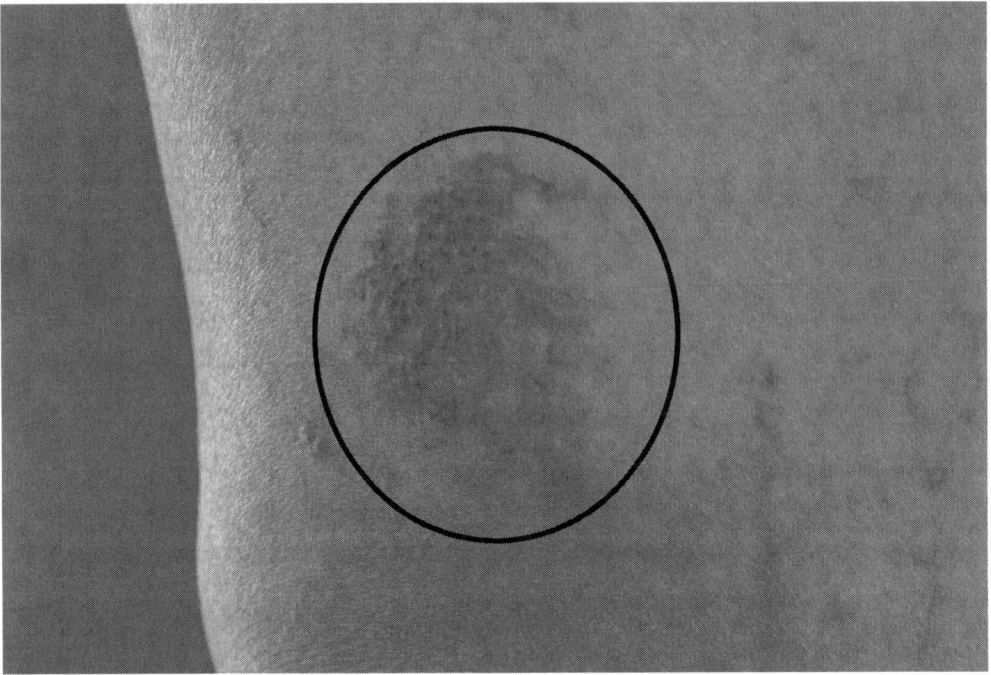

Fig. 8-12. These veins also protrude but again, these are not varicose veins and they SHOULD be bled. Prick two or three. Keep squeezing blood out and wiping with an alcohol swab to keep the blood flowing until it is done. Such bleeding is unlikely to result in bruising; to the contrary this could also be considered "cosmetic bleeding" as this patch will be more faint afterwards. *Full-color picture at www.chinesebloodletting.com.*

Bleeding legs

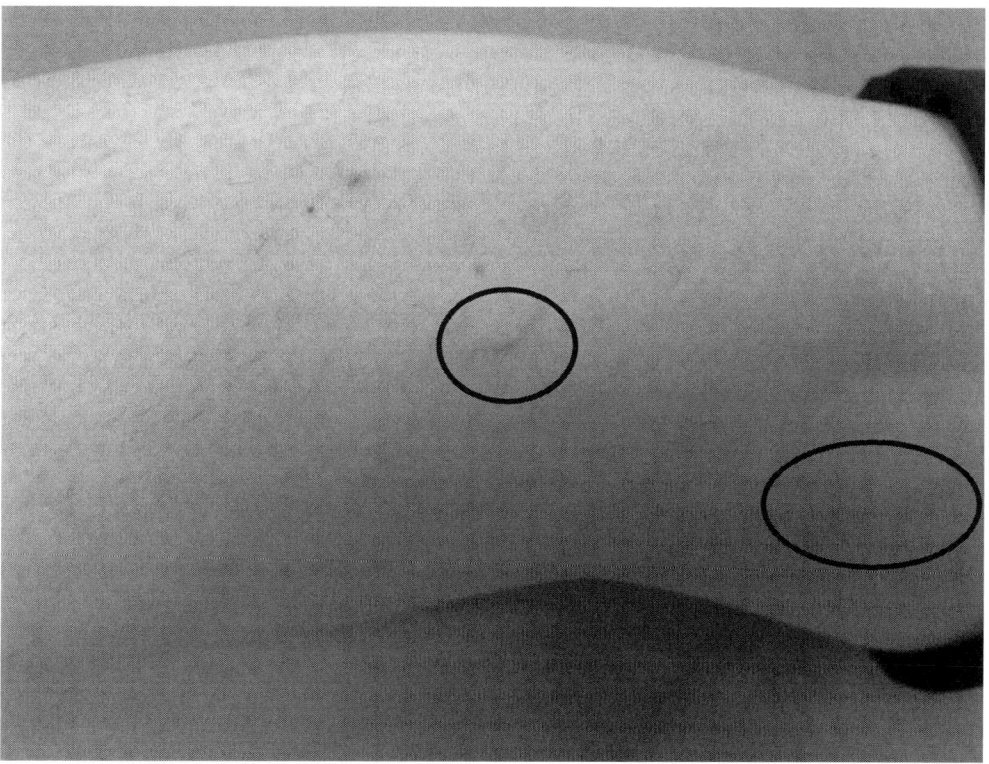

Fig. 8-13. Often you will not find any prominent dark veins—the most you will find is thin veins such as these. Nevertheless, bleeding them can have profound effects, even if just a small amount of blood is released. *Full-color picture at www.chinese-bloodletting.com.*

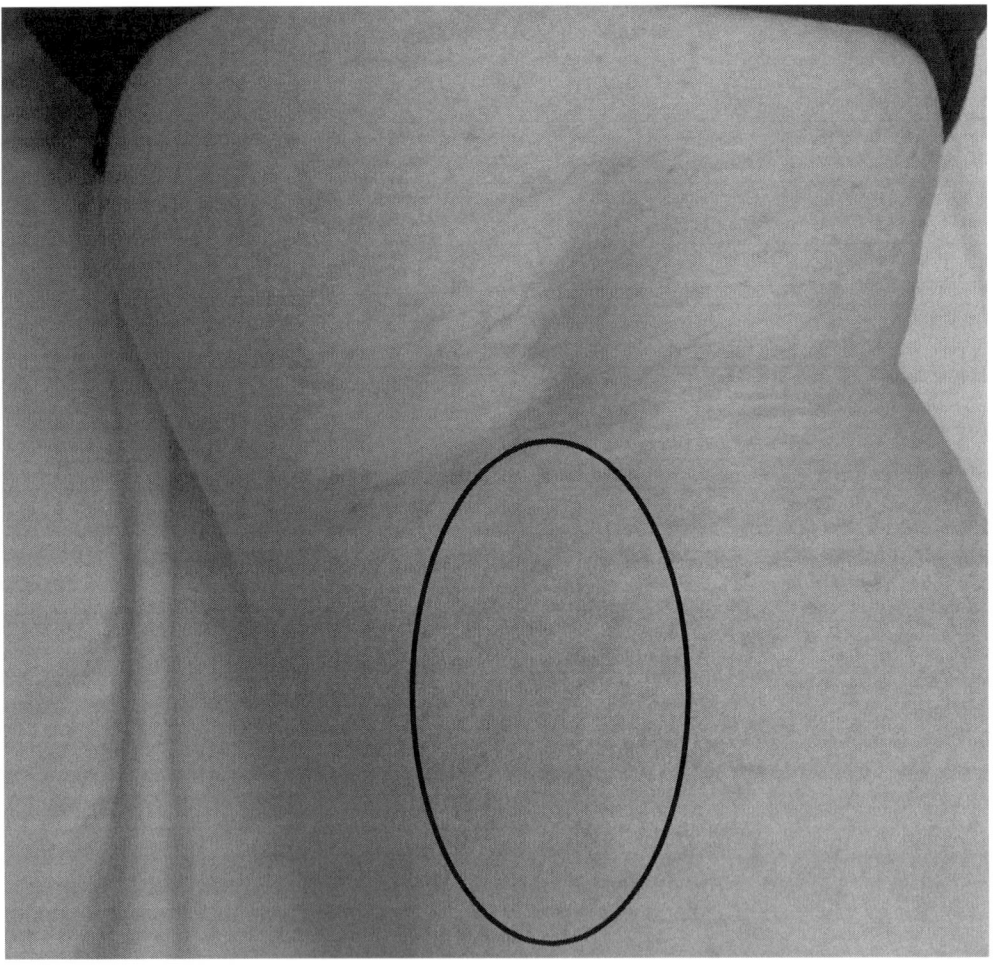

Fig. 8-14. Sometimes the only veins you find are so faint you can hardly see them—they are still good to bleed. *Full-color picture at www.chinesebloodletting.com.*

Bleeding legs

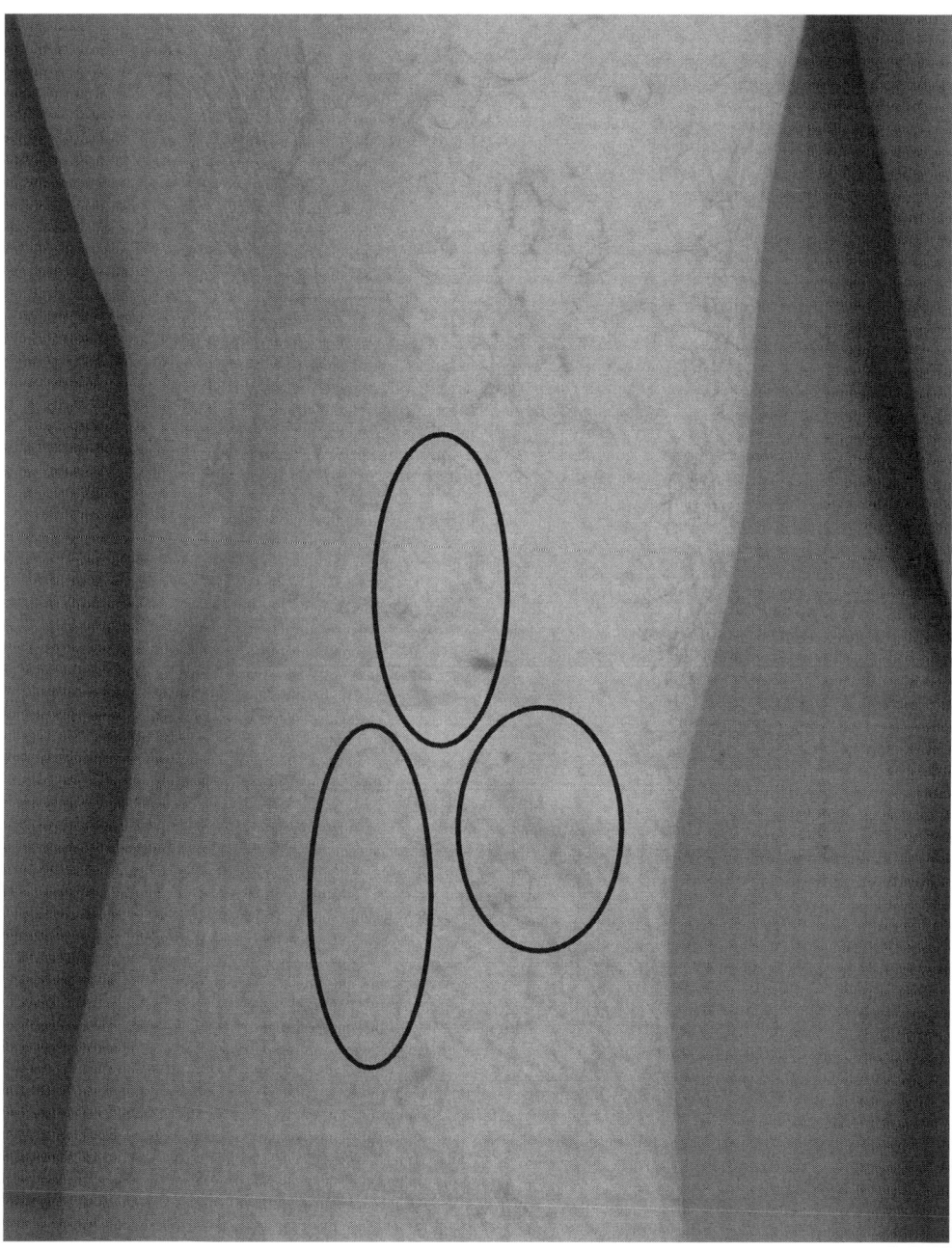

Fig. 8-15. These veins are faint but they are clearly visible and therefore good to bleed if there seems any reason to do so—indications such as sciatica, abdominal pain, occipital headache, hemorrhoids and many more. *Full-color picture at www. chinesebloodletting.com.*

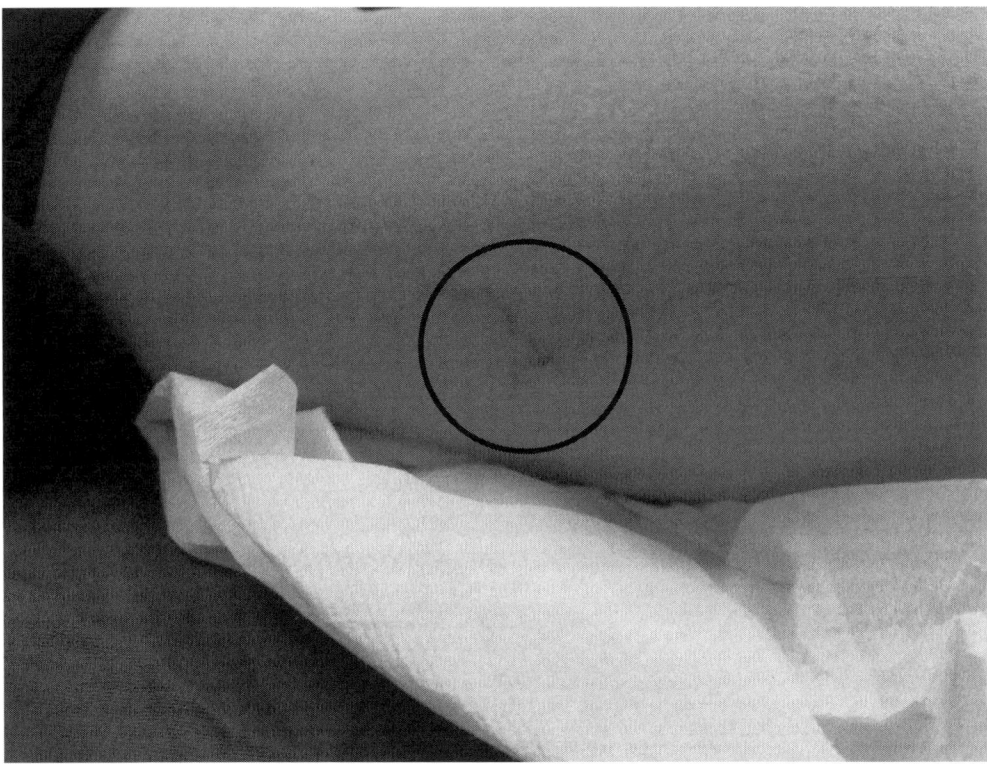

Fig. 8-16. This patient presented with an occipital migraine. Upon inspection, this vein, just proximal to GB36, was the only visible vein on her leg. Even though it is outside of the Tung "occipital region," I bled it and the patient's migraine immediately reduced 80%. This is a good example of "Bleed what you see, wherever it is."
Full-color picture at www.chinesebloodletting.com.

Bleeding legs

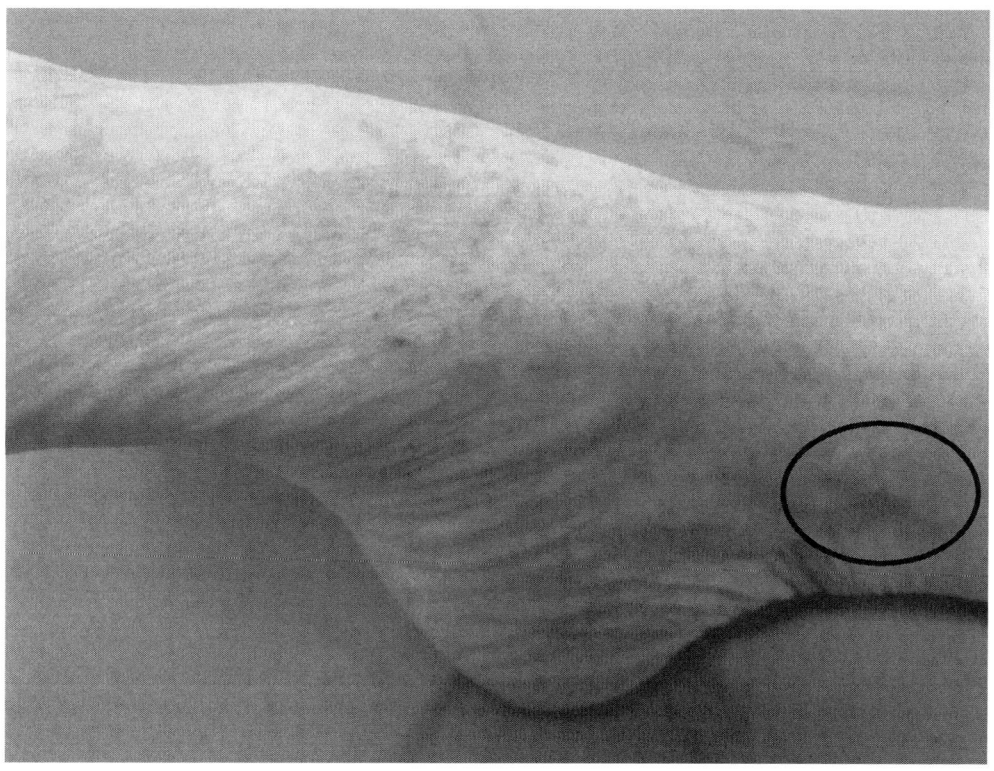

Fig. 8-17. This protruding vein should not be bled. The dark, flat veins on the ankle, however, can be bled. *Full-color picture at www.chinesebloodletting.com.*

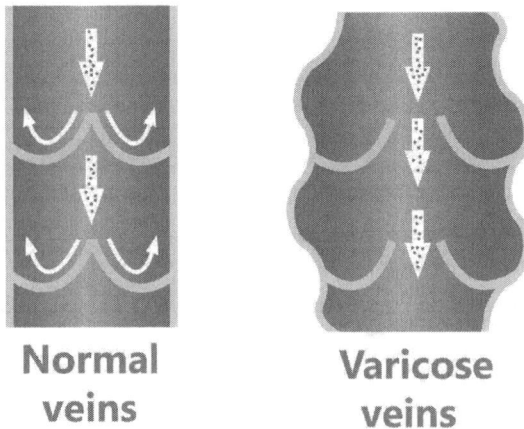

Fig. 8-18. Healthy veins in the legs have valves that prevent gravity from causing "backflow" of blood. In varicose veins, those valves are diseased and no longer function. You should never bleed varicose veins themselves, but you can and should bleed flat, visible veins (especially dark ones if any are present) on the same leg. This is an effective treatment for varicose veins and will cause them to shrink.

Bleeding legs

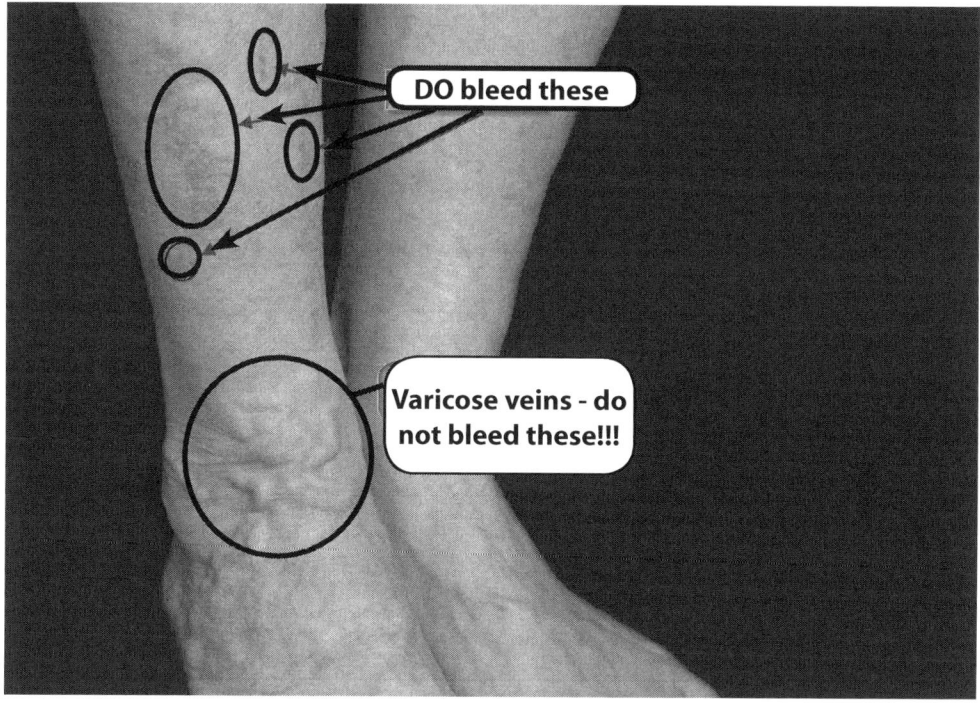

Fig. 8-19. Do NOT bleed the varicose veins circled in this picture at the woman's right ankle. However, you can and should bleed the dark, flat veins circled above the ankle. *Full-color picture at www.chinesebloodletting.com.*

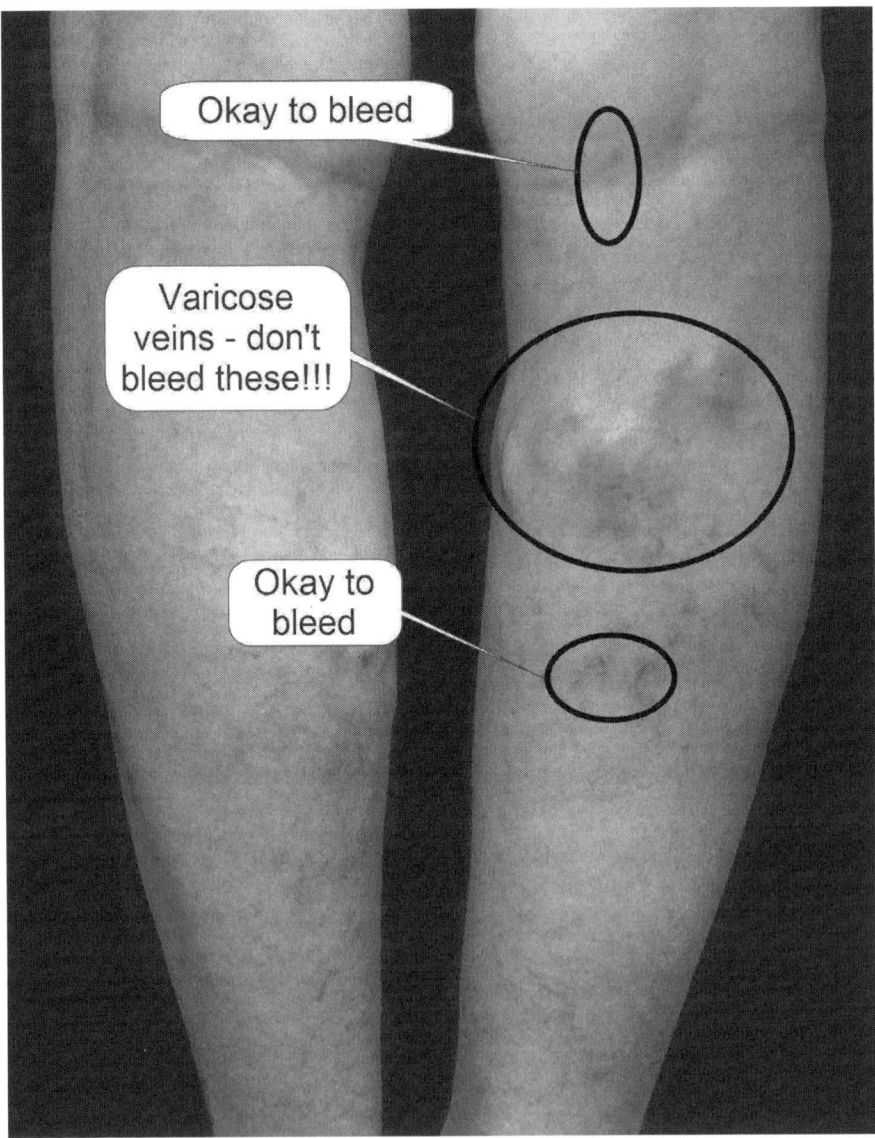

Fig. 8-20. Avoid bleeding the bulging varicose veins, but DO bleed flat, visible veins in the same leg. *Full-color picture at www.chinesebloodletting.com.*

Bleeding legs

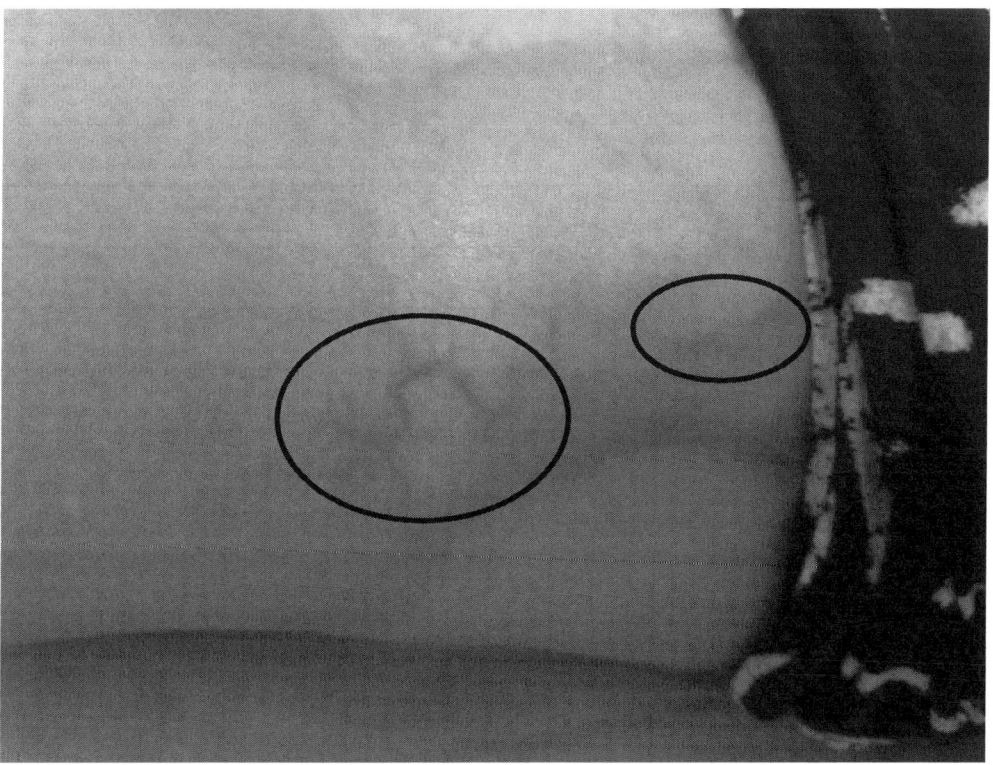

Fig. 8-21. This woman presented with stubborn occipital headaches and—conveniently—prominent dark veins right in her Master Tung "occipital region." The headaches resolved after bleeding twice—once within the circles, and once wet-cupping her back (B points tender to palpation just lateral to the spine at approximately T9-T10). *Full-color picture at www.chinesebloodletting.com.*

Positioning the patient

Chinese practitioners typically have patients sit or stand for bloodletting. In this position gravity helps the blood to flow, so it is the best for obtaining the greatest amount of blood.

Based on what we now know about vasovagal reactions and the risks of fainting, however, I consider bleeding a patient while standing to be unacceptably risky. Please see the section "Fainting" on page 44.

To sum up the risk, a small percentage of patients have vasovagal reactions to blood withdrawal and can feel faint or can actually faint. All it would take is one incident of a patient fainting from a standing position, and the result could be serious injury to the patient and devastating legal and financial implications for your practice. The probability of fainting is far less if the patient is lying down. And in the unlikely event someone did faint while lying down, no harm would come of it.

Also, you need to consider what the patient can see when you position them. A primary reason patients faint during phlebotomy is the sight of blood. When patients are lying face down they see nothing. Even lying face up they don't see what you are doing unless they make a point of sitting up to look.

Supplies/tools for bleeding legs

Bleeding needles

Remember that bleeding legs is venous bleeding. In other words, you find veins using visual inspection and bleed them directly. Unlike bleeding the back, palpation is unnecessary.

Diabetic lancets are inadequate for bleeding veins in legs, you should rather use hypodermic needles. Blood is flowing directly from a vein, so cupping is unnecessary.

Following is a description of needles used for bleeding veins, including hypodermic needles. This is what I recommend, and what I use in my own practice.

Hypodermic needles

The preferred instrument for bleeding veins in legs is hypodermic needles. In the US you can buy the McKesson and BD brands, both of which are regulated and manufactured to the highest standards, and used in clinics and hospitals.

In addition, hypodermic needles are coated with a thin coating of medical silicone, which makes them even more comfortable for patients. Piercing needles are not coated with silicone and thus can be more painful.

Finally—and surprisingly—hypodermic needles are less expensive than piercing needles.

Both piercing needles and hypodermic needles are available in different gauges. My preferred diameter for bleeding needles is 1.2mm. Be aware that the gauge numbers for piercing needles and hypodermic needles are not equivalent. A needle with the preferred diameter of 1.2mm is a 16 gauge piercing needle, but an 18 gauge hypodermic needle. My personal preference is an 18 gauge hypodermic needle. 20 gauge hypodermic needles work well too, and are preferable for novice bloodletters.

Three-edge needles

The classic instrument for Chinese bloodletting is the 3-edge needle. Master Tung and other Chinese practitioners constantly sharpened and cleaned their 3-edge needles, and used them over and over again.

Today, most states in the U.S. mandate single-use, pre-sterilized, disposable needles for acupuncture. Sharpening, sterilizing and re-using needles is not permitted by law.

You can buy single-use, pre-sterilized 3-edge needles. However, in my experience they are not sharp, and cause pain and discomfort for patients. I recommend against using them.

Piercing needles

Piercing needles are essentially cut-off hypodermic needles used by tattoo parlors for body piercing. They are razor-sharp and work well. You can order them from tattoo supply houses or from Amazon.

However, I no longer use them. The problem is that they often come in plain white boxes from China, with no labeling. There is no way of knowing who manufactured them. Often there is no lot number stamped on the needle packaging. So if ever there was a problem, you would not be able to trace the manufacturer, and you could conceivably be held legally responsible for failing to taking proper care in choosing your needles.

Piercing needles often come in plastic-bubble packaging, with a small styrofoam ball on the sharp tip to prevent them from piercing the plastic, which would compromise their sterility. However, these balls frequently come off in shipping, so it is difficult to be certain that the needle has not pierced the plastic and is still sterile. (See picture below) This is unacceptable—when inserting a needle, you cannot have any doubts about its sterility.

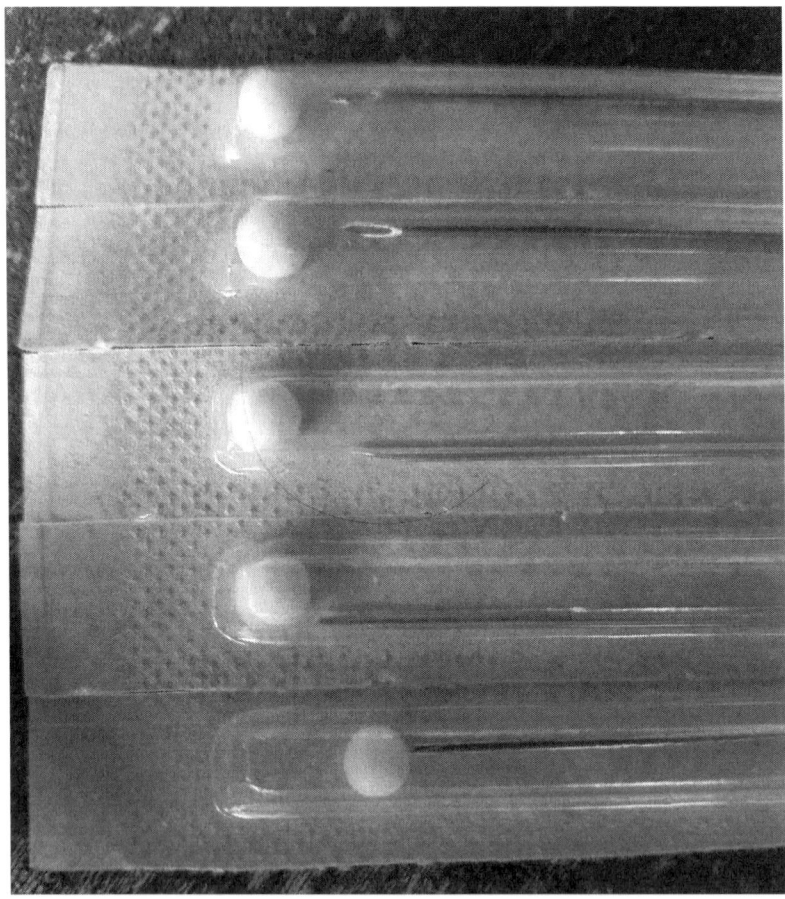

Fig. 8-22. Piercing needles ordered from Amazon and sent from China. You can see that in most of them the point has become separated from the protective styrofoam ball, possibly compromising the needle's sterility.

To maintain the highest standards of safety, quality, and sterility of your bleeding needles, I highly recommend the use of hypodermic needles. You can buy and use the same ones used in hospitals and clinics, eliminating any question about their quality or sterility.

Don't use diabetic lancets for bleeding legs!

It MAY be possible to bleed the veins in a patient's legs with diabetic lancets if the veins are extremely superficial. But for the most part, diabetic lancets produce poor results when used to bleed veins, as they don't go deep enough. Both you and your patient will likely end up annoyed and frustrated by your having to prick multiple times with little or no result.

Don't risk this happening to you. If you are going to bleed veins, do it right. Use an appropriate instrument, preferably a hypodermic needle.

Step-by-step instructions for bleeding legs

Bleeding legs means bleeding veins

When we bleed legs we are bleeding veins. The darker vein, the better—although you can obtain excellent clinical results bleeding even faint greenish veins.

Sometimes the only vein you can find is so faint, you're not sure if it's really there or if you're imagining it. The way to find out is to prick it. If blood flows out, you got a vein.

Since we are directly bleeding veins, there is no need to use a cup to encourage blood flow—the blood will flow adequately on its own. Also, we do not need to palpate, as we can see the veins we want to bleed. So instead of palpation being our guide to exactly where to bleed, our eyes are our guide. We bleed the veins we see, the darkest ones we can find. If we cannot find any dark veins, lighter ones will do.

The bleeding needle of choice is a hypodermic needle. I personally use 18 gauge or 20 gauge McKesson hypodermic needles; BD is another good brand.

Procedure for bleeding legs

As mentioned previously, I bleed legs with patients lying down on a massage table.

First, place an absorbent pad underneath the area to be bled. I'm currently using Attends brand Dri-Sorb underpads, 24" x 17" size (see Appendix I—supplies).

Next, set up a clean field by placing a few paper towels on a nearby surface. It is better to use a surface other than the table for this, to avoid the patient touching instruments with their leg if they change positions.

On your clean field, place the items you will need for bleeding veins. These include bleeding needles, cotton balls or gauze to wipe and absorb blood, packaged alcohol wipes, and bandages. Also have your sharps container nearby.

Put your gloves on and clean the area to be bled. Normally I use alcohol swabs for this, but if there is reason for greater caution I may use Betadine (povidone iodine). Always ask first if the patient is allergic to iodine before using. I sometimes use Betadine on or near the feet, since feet can harbor a lot of bacteria.

Following is the pricking technique in detail. For this we will assume a right-handed practitioner.

Place a cotton ball or gauze in your left hand. Then place a needle in your right hand, holding the shaft of the needle between your thumb and forefinger as in Fig. 8-23 below.

Bleeding legs

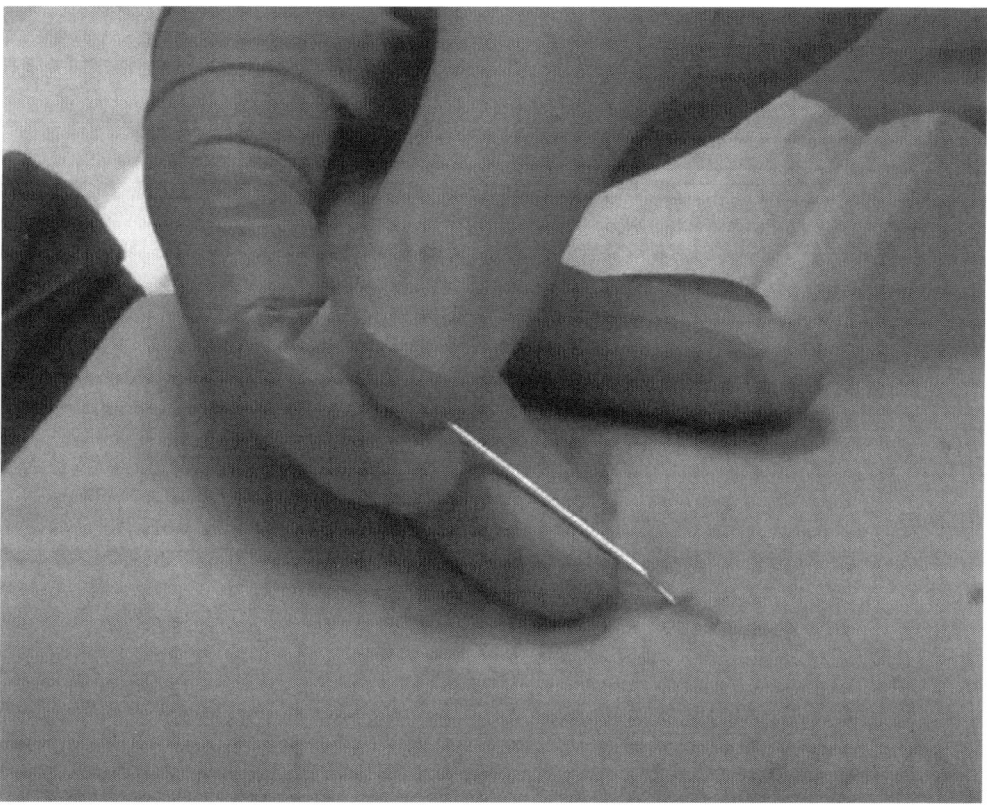

Fig. 8-23. Holding an 18g hypodermic needle with the plastic nib between thumb and forefinger, and the middle finger controlling the tip. This picture was taken a split second before pricking the vein with a quick "rolling" motion. *Full-color picture at www.chinesebloodletting.com.*

The Complete Guide to Chinese Medicine Bloodletting

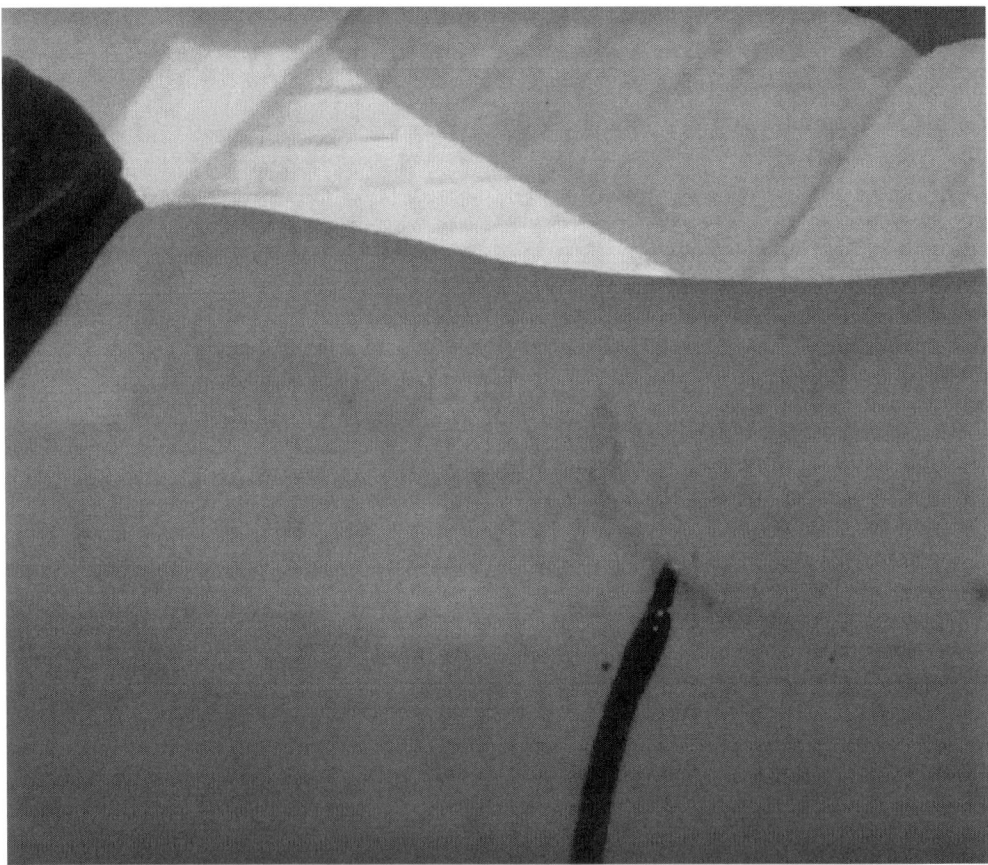

Fig. 8-24. A moment later, after pricking that vein. Note the dark color of the blood. This patient, Tasha, has interstitial cystitis and had come in for treatment of a flareup. Bleeding the UB40 or ST36/GB34 area almost never fails to bring her instant relief. See "Tasha's interstitial cystitis" on page 221. *Full-color picture at www.chinesebloodletting.com.*

Place your middle finger on the shaft near the point. This finger controls the tip and will determine how deep the needle can go. Adjust the depth based on the type of vein. If it is a very superficial purple vein, a millimeter or two will do. If it is a faint green vein, you will need to go slightly deeper.

Hold the point directly on the vein, bevel up. Make a mental note that blood may spurt, so you will not panic to cover it with your left hand, possibly sticking yourself accidentally. You can depress the skin a little with the needle if you like.

Roll the needle to make a quick insertion. If that seems clumsy you can simply stick it quickly.

IMMEDIATELY pull your right hand away and discard the needle in a sharps container.

When it looks as though the flow of blood is slowing, you can gently squeeze around the puncture to encourage further flow. Ideally you want to let the blood keep flowing until it stops on its own. You can keep it flowing longer by occasionally swabbing with an alcohol swab, which will temporarily prevent a clot from forming.

Watch to see if a bruise is forming. If so, apply firm but gentle pressure to the puncture for 2 minutes or so with clean cotton or gauze. The purpose of this is to stop blood from flowing out of the vein long enough so hemostasis may form at the vein. This may not completely prevent bruising, but is effective at minimizing it.

After you remove pressure, watch the puncture for at least 10 seconds to make sure the internal bleeding has stopped and the bruise is not continuing to form.

Gauze is better than cotton for applying pressure on the puncture, as fibers from cotton may become embedded in the blood clot covering the puncture. When you remove the cotton, that may disturb the clot and re-open the puncture, causing it to bleed again. For that reason, phlebotomy guidelines discourage the use of cotton balls and encourage the use of gauze.

Does the gauze or cotton have to be sterile? No. According to phlebotomy guidelines, there are only three sterile aspects of phlebotomy—the alcohol swab, the needle, and the bandage. Other aspects need not be sterile. Still, surveys show that approximately a third of phlebotomists use sterile gauze to apply pressure to puncture sites.

I also use sterile gauze. This is really due to the way they come packaged. Sterile gauze pads come individually packaged so their sterility at the time of use is guaranteed. Non-sterile gauze pads do not come individually packaged so as a practical matter, it is more difficult to guarantee their cleanliness. Sterile gauze pads are not expensive so on balance, I recommend their use.

After a clot has formed, clean the blood off the patient's skin, avoiding direct contact with the puncture so as not to disturb the clot. You can use alcohol-soaked cotton or cotton wipes. Hydrogen peroxide (3%) works better than alcohol to remove dried blood from skin, and is a disinfectant as well.

Finally, apply a bandage to cover the puncture. I tell patients to keep it dry for the next several hours, and not to remove the bandage for at least that much time. However, they should not wait too long to take the bandage off, as the adhesive can harden and it can become difficult to remove.

Work your way from bottom up, not top down

If you are planning on bleeding two points in a vertical line, be sure to bleed the bottom one first. If you bleed the top one first, blood will cover the lower point and make it difficult to see and bleed.

How effective will it be? How to gauge probable efficacy

What to look for before bleeding

Recall from the previous chapter that when bleeding the upper back, palpation will tell you how likely it is that bleeding will be effective. The more tender to palpation the point you find, the greater the probability that bleeding will be effective.

When bleeding legs however, remember that your eyes are your guide, not your fingers. You are looking for suitable veins to bleed. Dark purple is the color of blood stasis, and veins such as those pictured in Fig. 8-25 below are a manifestation of significant blood stasis. Finding and bleeding such veins is very likely to benefit your patient.

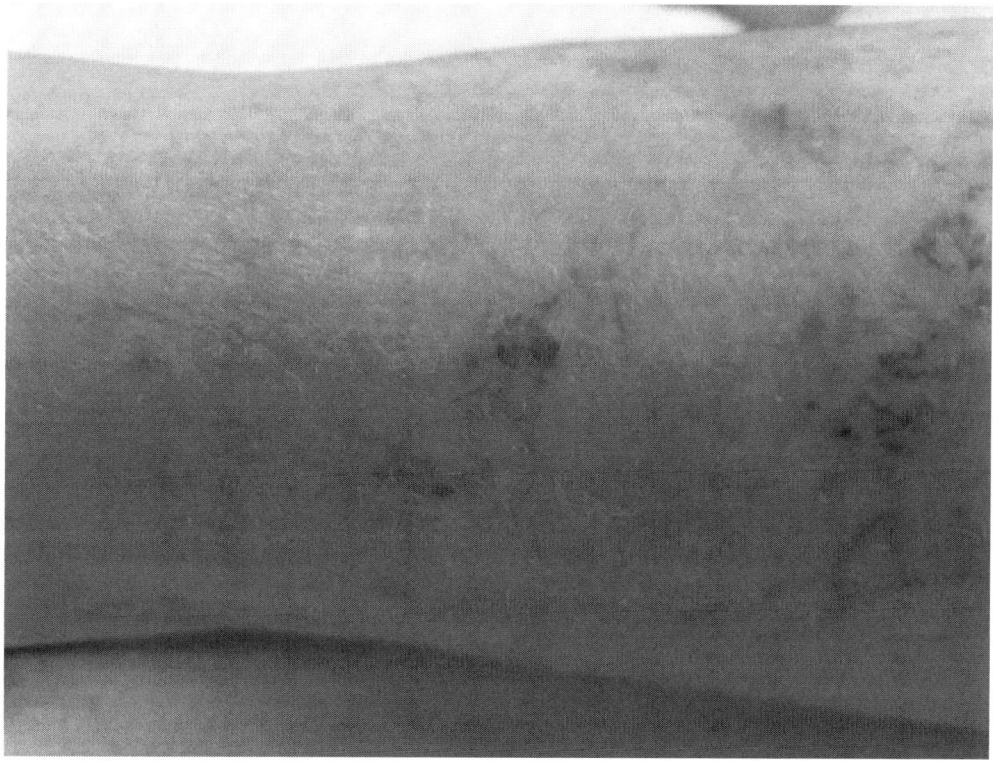

Fig. 8-25. These dark veins are a clear indication of blood stasis; it is good to bleed them. *Full-color picture at www.chinesebloodletting.com.*

What to look for during bleeding

Occasionally blood will spurt when you prick a vein. Usually it's just an initial spurt and lasts no more than a second, but rarely it can spurt for longer. Either way, it's a good sign. It means that blood was under pressure, which is an indication of blood stasis.

The pressure is an indication of a blockage or impediment to blood flow downstream. Just as a dam causes water pressure to rise upstream, blood stasis causes venous pressure to rise upstream. Blood spurting is a sign of that increased pressure.

In Western terms, that pressure is a likely indicator of inflammation that is narrowing the vein downstream, like stepping on a garden hose. That is painful. The spurting indicates the pressure is being relieved, likely with accompanying relief of pain.

If the blood comes out dark, that is an indication of blood stasis and a strong indicator of probable success. Ideally the blood will come out dark at first, then turn bright red as the static blood is evacuated and replaced with fresh, circulating blood. This is particularly true of venous bleeding, where the color of blood is a reliable sign of whether the bleeding will be effective or not. Color is also an indicator with capillary bleeding, but is an even more clear sign with venous bleeding.

Chapter 9

Bleeding ears

Bleeding ears is as quick, easy, and safe as any technique in Chinese medicine. For many indications it is also amazingly effective. If the only type of bleeding you ever do in your practice is bleeding ears, it will still tremendously enhance your clinical results and produce many "miracles."

Any time a patient comes in with a headache, trigeminal neuralgia, dental pain, problems of vision or around the eyes, post- mastectomy pain or discomfort, pain/discomfort in the upper limbs—especially any pain pattern that seems to indicate a pinched nerve—the first thing I will do is to bleed the ear. For anxiety, depression, and insomnia I will almost always bleed the ear as well.

List of indications for bleeding ears

Following is a partial list of conditions for which I have successfully bled ears:

- Acne
- Anxiety
- Arm pain/numbness
- Axillary sweat glands, blocked
- Carpal tunnel syndrome
- Conjunctivitis
- Dental pain

- Depression
- Ear pain
- Fever
- Hand pain/numbness
- Headache
- Hypertension
- Insomnia
- Lymph node removal (post-surgical pain/discomfort due to axillary lymph node removal)
- Mastectomy pain (post-mastectomy syndrome)
- Migraine
- Neck pain
- Optic neuritis
- Palpitations
- Pharyngitis
- Pruritis
- Ptosis
- Ribcage pain, including pain of ankylosing spondylitis
- Shoulder pain
- Stye
- Sweaty palms (hyperhidrosis)
- TMJ
- Tonsillitis
- Trigeminal neuralgia
- Spasming above the eye

Where to bleed ears

Where on the ear should you bleed? Generally I just bleed the apex, but you can also bleed any capillaries or small veins you find, particularly behind the ear.

Master Tung describes two points to be bled for ears. The first is 99.07, which is on the back of the ear. Look for a tiny blue vein there and prick it.

The second "point" to bleed is 99.08, which is actually a "three-point unit" and consists of 99.08-1, 99.08-2, and 99.08-3, as shown in Fig. 9-1 below.

Weh-Chieh Young recommends bleeding two points when bleeding the ear—the apex (99.08-1) and one additional point of your choice—either the most posterior point on the ear helix (99.08-2) or the bottom of the lobe (99.08-3). He also mentions the option of bleeding the blue vein at the back of the ear.[17]

But personally I like to keep it simple—in most cases I just bleed the ear apex. If ear bleeding is going to work, I find this is adequate to do the job. If necessary, I will poke more than once to get an adequate amount of blood—at least 5 good drops. Sometimes I will also bleed posterior to 99.08-1, towards 99.08-2

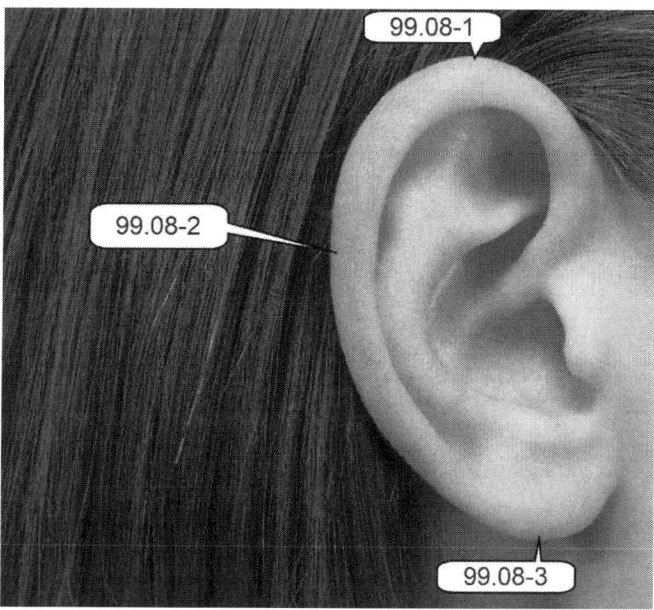

Fig. 9-1.

Positioning the patient—danger of fainting

I used to have patients sit on a stool when bleeding their ears. The patient was on my left, while a table with bleeding supplies was on my right. If I needed to bleed both ears, I could simply bleed one ear, then have the patient swivel 180 degrees and bleed the other ear.

However, a few years ago a patient fainted when I bled her ear. There was no warning—she had not been nervous about it in the least. But I bled one ear and before I knew what was happening, she slumped off the stool and fell to the floor unconscious. She had started to say she felt woozy, but I was unable to catch her in time.

We were both very lucky as she was unhurt. But it served as a warning, and I have changed my procedures since then. When I bleed someone's ears now, I have them sit in a chair that is sturdy and has a slightly reclining position so if they do faint, they won't go anywhere. If they are particularly large, infirm or have a known history of fainting during blood withdrawal, I will have them lie down to bleed their ear.

If a patient is sitting and tells you he or she is starting to feel faint, assume that they WILL faint and take steps to revive them immediately. It is typical for patients to say they feel faint, then assure you they'll be okay, and then suddenly lose consciousness.

I always have an instant chemical cold-pack at hand now. You simply squeeze the pack where indicated in order to activate the chemicals inside, which makes the pack instantly cold. Slip the cold pack behind the patient's neck, which will help to revive them.

Please also see the section "Fainting" on page 44.

Supplies/tools for bleeding ears

Lancets

My preferred lancet for bleeding ears is a 21 gauge manual lancet. In the U.S. you cannot find these in drugstores, where the thickest lancets are usually 26 gauge (the higher the gauge, the thinner the lancet). You have to order 21g lancets online.

If you are unable to obtain 21g lancets, you can use lancets of a higher gauge. You will have to prick a few more times though.

You can also bleed ears using the 17g safety lancets that are recommended in this book for bleeding the back. But for my purposes these work a little TOO well. They allow you to get an adequate amount of blood all right, but then it can take several minutes of applying pressure with a q-tip or gauze on the puncture site to get the bleeding to stop completely. That is a long time in a busy practice.

I find the 21g lancets give just the right balance—you can get enough blood by squeezing it out drop by drop, but when you stop squeezing, the blood flow is usually easy to stop.

Other supplies

In addition to lancets, you will also need:
- Alcohol swabs
- Cotton balls, q-tips or gauze to wipe blood and stop bleeding
- Medical gloves

Step-by-step instructions for bleeding ears

As noted earlier, I usually have patients sit in a chair to bleed ears.

First, prepare your clean field, and place cotton balls, q-tips and/or sterile gauze on it. Also place a few lancets

- Put on medical gloves.
- Swab the ear or ears you are going to bleed.
- Determine where you are going to prick. Most often I just prick the apex, but sometimes I prick a few additional points as well (see "Where to bleed ears," above).
- Pinch up the skin so you can prick just skin and avoid pricking the cartilage. Pricking the cartilage would not cause a problem, but the less tissue affected, the better.
- Quickly prick the pinched-up skin with your lancet, and note how much blood comes out. If you get a few drops quickly, that's good. If nothing or very little comes out, prick again nearby.
- Discard the lancet into a sharps container. Squeeze out blood from the ear and wipe with your gauze, cotton ball or q-tip. Continue until

you've gotten 5-20 good drops of blood.

- You can keep squeezing out blood as long as you wish. When you are done, hold your gauze, cotton ball or q-tip on the puncture(s) until it stops.

To massage ears before bleeding or not?

Many practitioners massage ears for a few minutes before bleeding to bring blood to the area. There is nothing wrong with this practice, and it does result in more blood.

Personally however I don't do it, as I haven't found it necessary. It also takes more time, and I see a lot of patients so time is of the essence. Finally, massaging the ears makes it seem as though bleeding them is more of a "production" than simply pricking and squeezing. This is the opposite of the impression I am trying to make, which is that pricking the ears and getting a few drops of blood is no big deal.

The diagnostic value of bleeding ears

Bleeding ears is both therapeutic and diagnostic. Diagnostic, because if the patient does experience some relief, you know for certain that this is a blood stasis issue and further bleeding is warranted.

If, however, the patient experiences zero relief after bleeding the ear, I put bleeding aside for the time being and try other approaches.

For this reason, it is important to get a clear baseline before bleeding. Tell your patient that you will want to know if there is any change when you are done, so please get a good sense of how the pain is now. If there is any movement that provokes the pain, have your patient do it so they can compare after bleeding.

If an unusually large amount of blood comes out after pricking the ear, that is usually associated with a good response.

The converse, however, is not true. Getting a very small amount of blood does not necessarily mean that bleeding will be ineffective.

All this assumes, of course, that you are bleeding for an indication known to respond to bleeding ears. For example, one would not expect knee pain to respond to ear bleeding—in that case, failure to respond would not be diagnostic.

Chapter 10

Additional areas to bleed

Bleeding arms

Bleeding arms usually means bleeding veins in the cubital fossa, such as those pictured below. The instruments and techniques are the same as for bleeding veins in the leg.

To be honest, the cubital fossa is not my favorite place to bleed. Veins there can be faint and difficult to find. It is not difficult to avoid hitting an artery or nerve, but doing so does require a little more care than bleeding other parts of the body

But the main reason that bleeding veins in the cubital fossa can be unpleasant is that these veins have a nasty tendency to bruise. Often I prick a vein there and as soon as the blood starts coming out, I see a greenish mound start to form around the puncture. This is blood extravasating into surrounding tissue, and a sure sign of an impending bruise. The only thing one can do at that point is to apply firm pressure for a few minutes using gauze. This will minimize the bruise, but will not eliminate it completely.

Nevertheless, bleeding veins in the cubital fossa is an important tool in the bleeding arsenal, particularly for stubborn problems of the upper limb such as frozen shoulder.

Sometimes, a vein will protrude right at the cubital fossa but if you follow it distally or proximally, it will become flat with the patient's skin. Better to bleed where it is flat, as it is less likely to bruise there.

Good light is important. Oftentimes, all you will see is a trace that is so faint, you will not be sure if it is a vein or if you're imagining it. If you think you see one, it's probably there.

For positioning—I find it easiest to have patients lie supine. That way I can put an impermeable pad under the arms, which makes cleanup easy. Also, most patients don't want to see what you're doing, and in this position they can't see the procedure unless they make a special effort and lift their heads.

Note that the brachial artery lies deep to PC3. You can find the exact location by palpating for a pulse. Caution is warranted if you are bleeding a vein that lies superficial to it. It should not be difficult to go just deep enough with your needle to prick the vein, avoiding the artery which lies much deeper. If in doubt, simply avoid bleeding where there is a pulse.

For bleeding veins in the cubital fossa, use the same instrument (hypodermic needle) and follow the same procedure as found in Chapter 8, "Bleeding legs."

What we can learn from phlebotomy about safely bleeding the cubital fossa.

Most blood draws are from veins in the cubital fossa, so we can learn much from phlebotomy about the risks of drawing blood from these veins, and about how to avoid problems.

The most common reason for phlebotomy-related lawsuits is nerve damage.

There are two possible causes of nerve damage during phlebotomy. The first is direct contact of a needle with the nerve. Phlebotomists are taught to go in at an angle of 15 to 30 degrees. If the angle is higher, it is easy to go too deep and injure a nerve.

This should never be a problem for acupuncturists performing bloodletting, as we are going in more shallowly, no more than a few mm, just pricking the top of the vein. Still, one cannot be careless here.

The other cause of nerve damage is a subcutaneous hemorrhage (hematoma, or bruise) from a vein or artery that continues bleeding into surrounding tissue. In rare cases, hematomas can become so large and extensive that they cause compartment syndrome and put pressure on a nerve, causing permanent damage.

Additional areas to bleed

This is why phlebotomists are taught to observe a puncture site for 10 seconds before placing a bandage on it—to make certain a bruise is not continuing to form, which would indicate continuing seepage of blood out of the vein (or artery) and into subcutaneous tissue.

If there is continued formation of a bruise, the phlebotomist should apply pressure on the puncture site for at least 2 minutes using clean or sterile gauze (5 minutes in the case of an artery puncture). This stops the blood flow and allows hemostasis to form at the vein, stopping the flow of blood out of the vein.

Almost all nerve injuries result from needling the basilic vein, which lies on the ulnar side of the cubital fossa. The basilic vein is close to both the median nerve and the brachial artery.

For that reason, phlebotomists are taught to draw blood from the basilic vein ONLY as a last resort, if no other vein will give satisfactory results.

Phlebotomists are also taught to palpate for a pulse if choosing a vein on the ulnar side of the cubital fossa, to make sure they are not over the brachial artery.

So to sum up, phlebotomists (and acupuncturists) can avoid problems when bleeding veins in the cubital fossa by:

- Preferring veins in the radial side of the cubital fossa (closer to LI11)
- Palpating for a pulse to locate the artery if bleeding on the ulnar side
- Watching for mounding (bruise formation) for at least ten seconds before applying a bandage, applying pressure for at least 2 minutes if mounding occurs, then checking again for another ten seconds when pressure is released.
- Acupuncturists can avoid direct contact with a nerve or artery by inserting the needle no more than a few mm, but that does not protect against subcutaneous hemorrhage (bruising) from a vein.

So in a nutshell—if you don't go in too deep, and if you apply pressure for sufficient time when you notice a bruise forming—you're safe. If you keep to the radial side of the cubital fossa (LI11 side), even better.

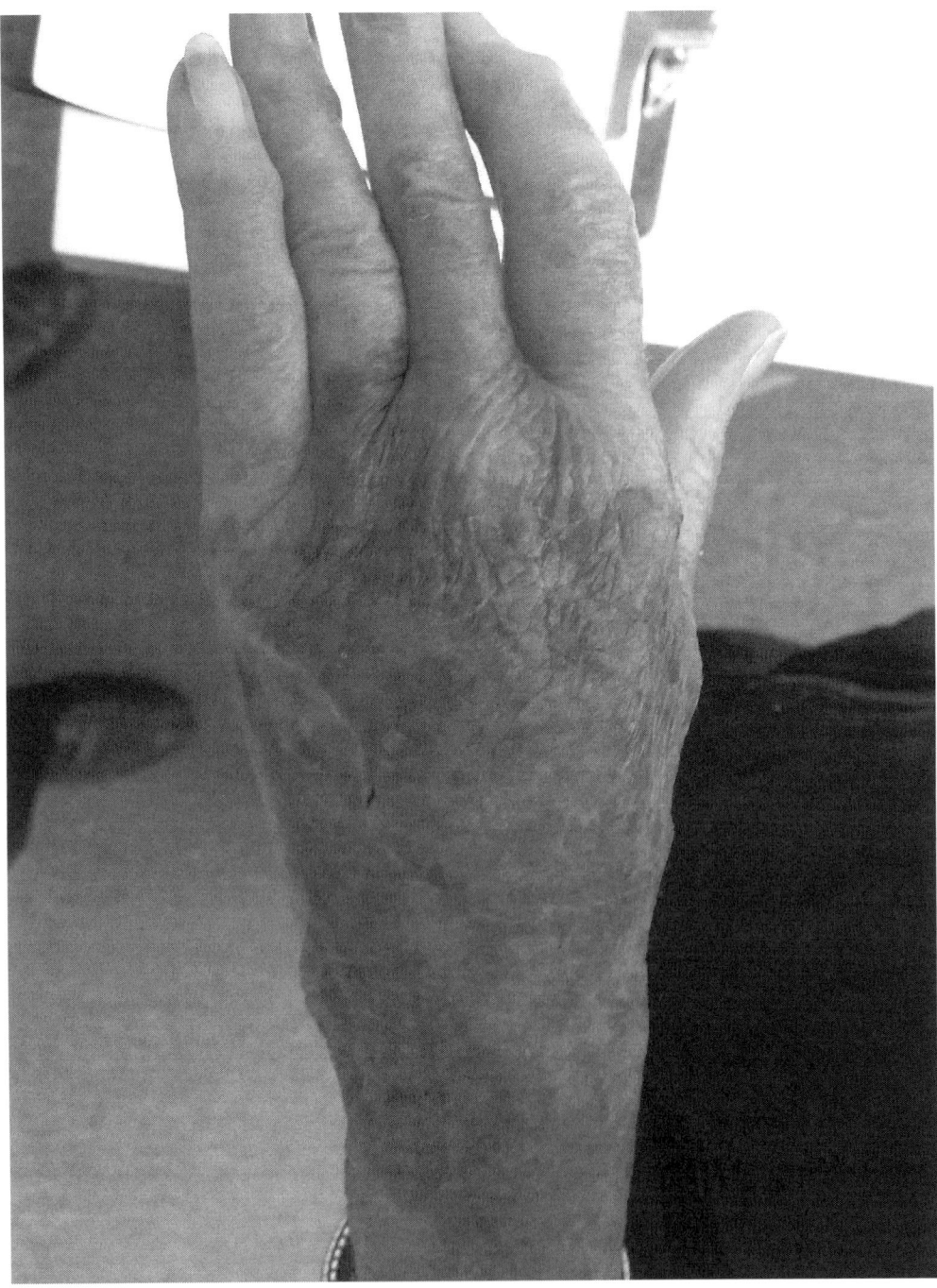

Fig. 10-1. Example of a large bruise caused by a punctured vein that bled subcutaneously. In this case nobody was at fault—the puncture was caused by a cat who

had been sitting in its owner's lap while both were sleeping. The phone rang, the owner and cat were startled and the cat dug in its claws, one of which pierced a vein with the result you see. Happily no lasting harm was done and the bruise resolved in a few weeks. *Full-color picture at www.chinesebloodletting.com.*

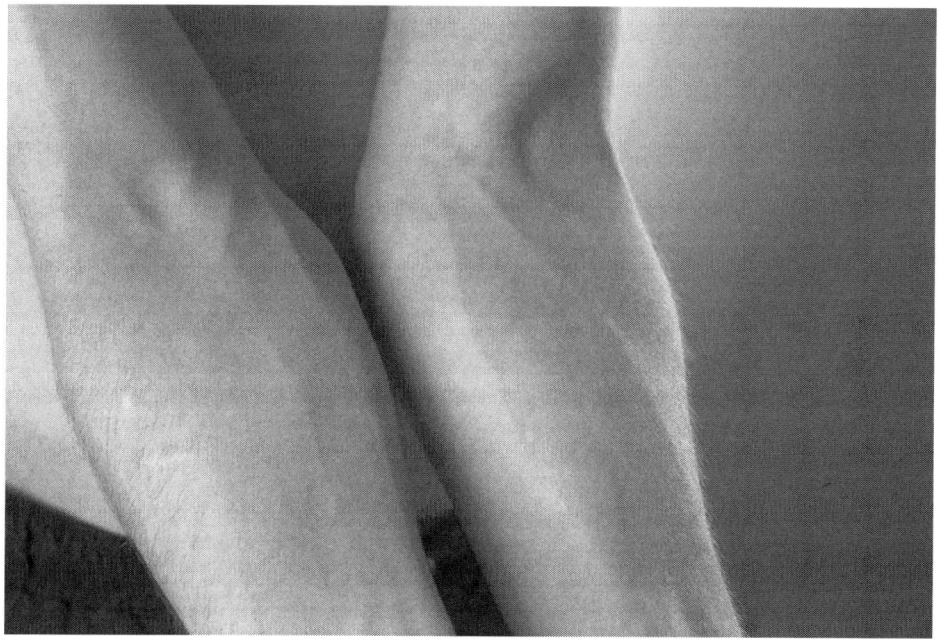

Fig. 10-2. Visible veins in the cubital fossa. It is better to avoid bleeding veins that protrude. If you see a protruding vein, simply follow it to where it is flat to the skin and prick there. *Full-color picture at www.chinesebloodletting.com.*

Predicting the efficacy of bleeding arms

Before bleeding arms, I have generally already bled ears, legs or upper back and gotten a positive response. That suggests that I am dealing with a blood stasis issue and—combined with the fact that this is an upper-limb problem—generally means that bleeding the cubital fossa will be successful.

Bleeding the Ventral Trunk (VT) areas

In Master Tung bloodletting there are 5 "points" or areas to bleed on the front of the neck, the chest, and the abdomen, numbered VT.01 to VT.05. VT stands for "Ventral Trunk." These points are always bled, never needled.

Bleeding the ventral trunk is less commonly done than bleeding the back. However, in certain situations it is the most effective approach.

The points on the anterior neck are VT.01, and are indicated for local issues such as tonsillitis, sore throat, thyroid issues such as goiter, and more.

To bleed these safely, simply pinch up the skin so you are sure to be bleeding skin only, and lance. I find the McKesson 17g safety lancets work well. You won't get a lot of blood which is fine—not much is needed for this to be effective. You don't cup of course—just squeeze out a bit of blood.

VT.02 to VT.05 are on the chest and abdomen. Their locations and indications for bleeding are listed below. These areas can be wet-cupped like areas on the back. The shallow penetration of the McKesson 17g safety lancets (2mm) makes them safe to use on almost every part of the body.

However, bleeding the abdomen can be tricky, especially in patients with a lot of abdominal fat. Not dangerous, just tricky. With fit, thin patients you can press on the abdomen with your safety lancets against the abdominal muscles and get good punctures. But the presence of soft adipose tissue in obese patients can make it difficult to press on anything solid and get an adequate puncture. For these patients you can pinch up some skin between thumb and forefinger and press your safety lancet firmly against the tissue you have pinched up.

Finally—it is important to use only GENTLE SUCTION when cupping the abdomen!!! I say this from personal experience, having once cupped the abdomen of a teenage girl using strong suction; the next morning the girl's mother called and told me she was in a lot of abdominal pain. Both mom and daughter were regular patients and not complainers, so I was worried. It took a few days to resolve and in the end no harm was done. But I have been cautious since.

VT.01 Hou'e Jiu (Throat Moth)

VT.01 is a "nine-point unit" as pictured in Fig. 10-3 below. The main point is directly over the Adams apple, with secondary points one cun above and one cun below. Less-important points are located 1.5 cun lateral to those three.

In reality, you only need that central point or a point nearby—the precise location is not important. Pinch the skin up so it is safely away from the underlying cartilage and prick once or twice with a lancet—safety lancets such as the McKesson 17g safety lancet are ideal. Do not cup in this area, simply squeezing out some blood is sufficient.

Bleeding VT.01 is effective for acute sore throat. In the case of tonsillitis, a test should be done for bacterial infection such as strep, and antibiotics pre-

Additional areas to bleed

scribed if appropriate. If the cause of tonsillitis is viral, bleeding VT.01 will relieve symptoms and speed healing. It can also be effective for thyroiditis and goiter.

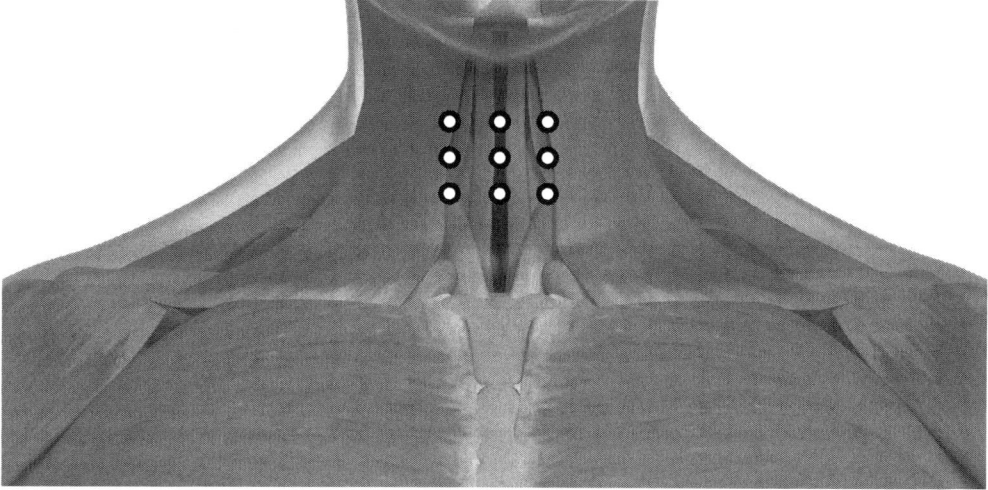

Fig. 10-3. VT.01

VT.02 Shi'er Hou (Twelve Monkeys)

VT.02 is a "12-point unit" as shown in Fig. 10-4 below. The first 3 points are located 1.3 cun below the clavicle on each side, and an additional 3 points are located 1.5 cun below those.

The classical indication for this area is scarlet fever. While the incidence of scarlet fever has dropped dramatically for over a century, the number of cases has been rising the past few years.

Palpate within the indicated area for a tender point on each side, and bleed by pinching up the skin and using a lancet or two, preferably a safety lancet such as the McKesson 17g. Pinch up the skin away from the chest for safety. You can simply squeeze out a little blood; cupping is probably not necessary.

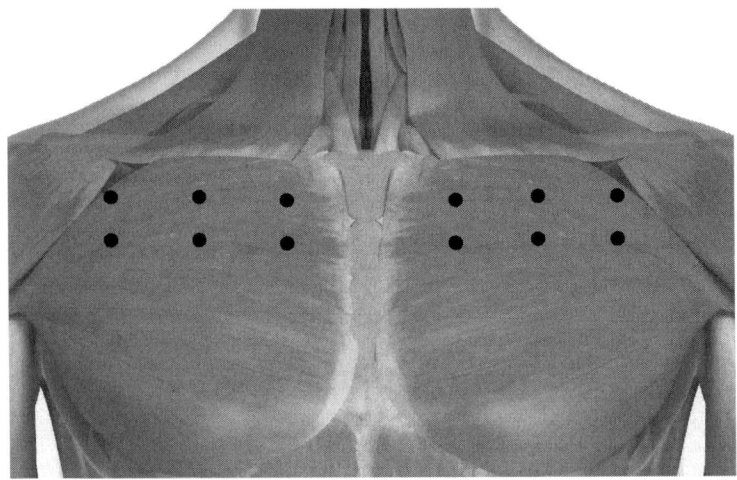

Fig. 10-4. VT.02

VT.03 Jin Wu (Metal Five)

This is a "5-point unit" with the most superior point in the center of the suprasternal fossa, and the next 4 points directly below at 1-cun intervals. You could also think of it simply as a 4-cun line beginning with the most superior point and extending down 4 cun.

Bleeding this area is indicated for the viral diseases of childhood that produce rashes such as measles and chicken pox. However, these are rarely seen any more. It is also indicated for various conditions of the trachea.

Palpate along this line for a point much more tender to palpation than others and if you find such a point, bleed it. If no such point is found, then there is no reason to bleed there.

It is best to bleed this area by pinching up the skin to lift it away from the underlying structures, and prick with a lancet. You can then cup gently, or just squeeze out a few good drops of blood.

Additional areas to bleed

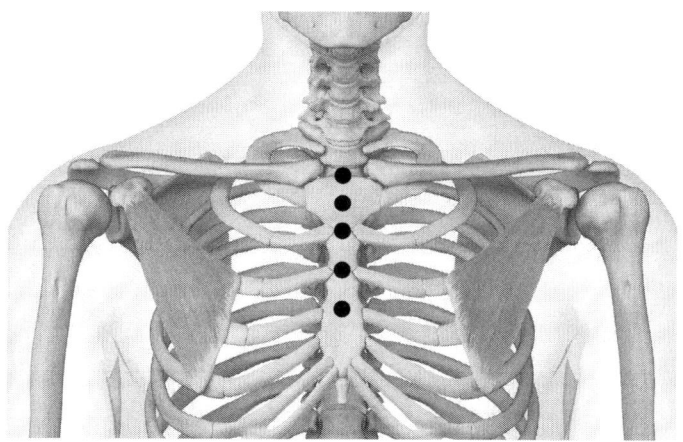

Fig. 10-5. VT.03

VT.04 Wei Mao Qi (Stomach Hair Seven)

VT.04 is a seven-point group consisting of the standard TCM points Ren 13, 14 and 15, and ST 19 and 20. You can also think of this as an area or zone.

This area is indicated for various acute gastric disorders. Palpate for a tender point and if you find one, bleed it by pinching up the skin and lancing. If you cup to encourage blood flow, you must do so gently. It is safer to just squeeze out a few good drops of blood.

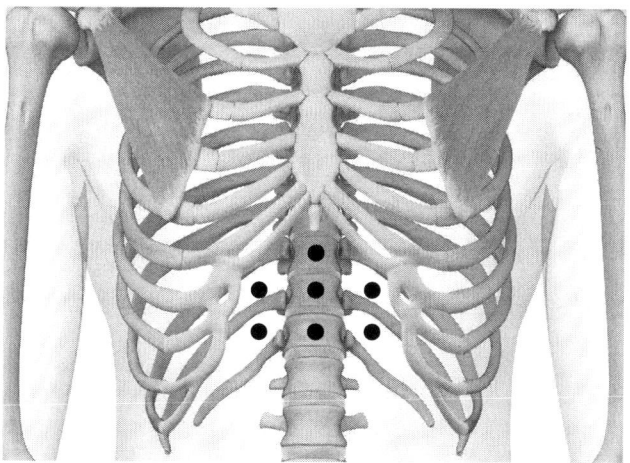

Fig. 10-6. VT.04

VT.05 Fu Chao'er Shi San (Bowel Nest 23)

This is a group of 23 points as shown in Fig. 10-7 below (the navel is not a point). Really this should be thought of as the entire area pictured, with the exception of the navel itself, which should NOT be bled.

Bleeding this area can be highly effective for various types of severe abdominal pain. It is particularly effective for pain of nephritis and other kidney conditions.

Palpate the area VERY gently to find a point that is significantly more tender to palpation than the surrounding area. Pinch up the skin, lance, and cup to encourage blood flow. Cupping in this area should be done gently, with just slight suction. Alternatively you can just squeeze out a few good drops of blood.

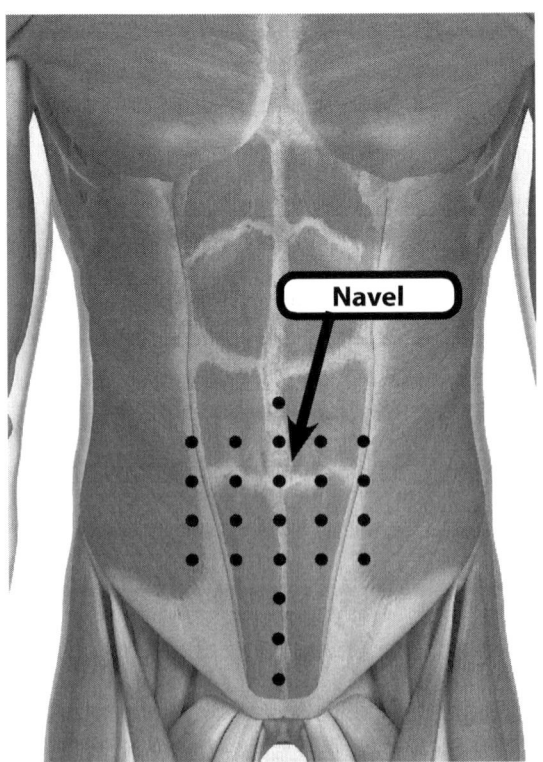

Fig. 10-7. VT.05

Bleeding the tip of the nose.

The point at the tip of the nose is DU 25 in the standard acupuncture numbering system, and 1010.12 in the Master Tung system. Bleed this point for rosacea, allergic rhinitis, and psychosis. Occasionally I have had good results with sinusitis.

Bleeding it is simple to do—just use a McKesson 17g safety lancet. One should be enough. You can squeeze gently to get a little additional blood.

While this point is easy to bleed, it is a bit awkward to squeeze out blood from it. In my experience patients are not that crazy about having this point bled, so I don't do it often.

Bleeding jing well points

Bleeding jing well points is indicated for stroke, especially during the acute phase. I personally have found bleeding these points on the affected side is also effective for Bell's palsy.

To bleed jing well points, I first place an absorbent, impermeable pad such as Chux on a massage table. I have the patient sit on a chair on one side of the table, and place his hand or hands to be bled on the pad. I sit on a stool on the opposite side.

To bleed jing-well points you will need:

- Lancets. The 17g McKesson/Acti-Lance safety lancets work well for this, as will any type of diabetic lancet
- Medical gloves
- Alcohol swabs
- Cotton balls or sterile gauze
- Bandages

Have the patient extend their hand palm-down on the pad or other surface. Put on gloves, and swab the points you are going to bleed with alcohol.

Using your lancet, lance the jing-well point. Squeeze out blood as long as it is flowing freely.

When you are done, hold a cotton ball, q-tip or gauze on the puncture until it stops bleeding. Place a bandage on it and tell the patient to remove it in 4-6 hours, and to keep it dry during that time.

Bleeding Tung point 11.26 Zhi Wu (Control Dirt)

This is a unique point unlike any others in the Master Tung bleeding tradition or any other tradition of which I am aware.

Bleeding 11.26 is specifically indicated for failure of a wound to heal, failure of a broken bone to join, or any other type of delayed healing. It is also bled for chronic skin ulcers that will not heal.

The name "Control Dirt" indicates that it is to be bled in cases of an infected wound as well. It can also be bled for abscesses. It is always bled ipsilateral to the problem.

Of course, patients with infections or non-healing wounds should be referred to a medical doctor. Often removal of pus and antibiotics are required for healing as well.

I have had consistently amazing results with bleeding point 11.26 in patients with longstanding injuries that had not healed despite the best interventions Western medicine had to offer. Two of my most amazing success stories with bleeding are described in Chapter 13—Case studies; "Katie's 3-year foot ordeal" on page 215, and "Sheila's heel that wouldn't heal" on page 216. Both cases resolved quickly after bleeding 11.26.

Tung point 11.26 is often described as a "three-point unit," but you can prick the vein anywhere along the proximal segment of the thumb as shown in Fig. 10-8.

To bleed 11.26, locate the blue vein on the proximal segment of the thumb. On most people it can be difficult to find but on patients for whom it should be bled, it is often engorged with blood. Perhaps that is how Master Tung's forebears discovered it.

Normally you should avoid bleeding bulging veins, but in the case of 11.26, it is okay to bleed this vein when it is engorged with blood. Such engorgement indicates that bleeding is appropriate.

Bleed this vein with a hypodermic needle such as an 18g or 20g needle. If you don't have any of those, it may be possible to bleed it with a manual diabetic lancet. You probably will not succeed in bleeding it with a spring-loaded safety lancet, as it is too difficult to aim with the required precision.

Additional areas to bleed

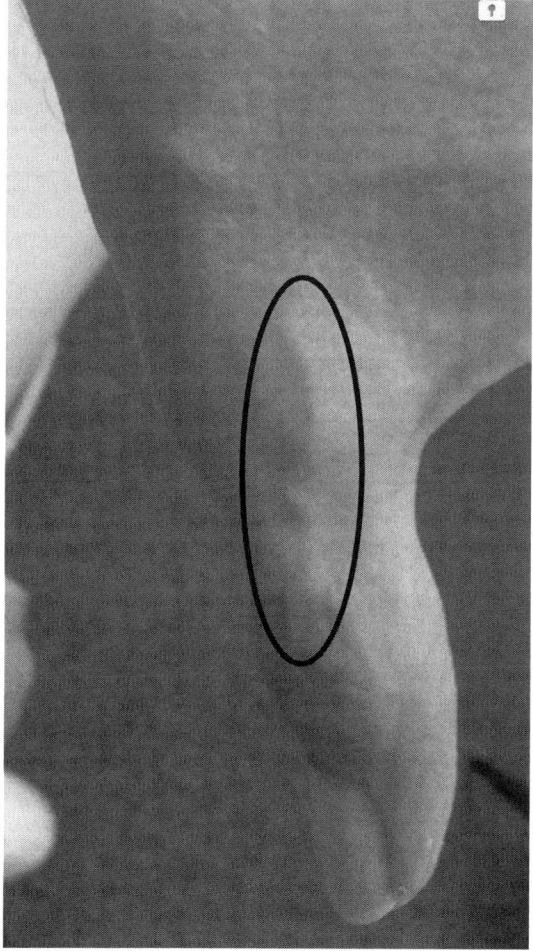

Fig. 10-8. Tung "point" 11.26 is sometimes shown as 3 points along the vein but in reality you can prick anywhere along the circled vein. Only one prick is necessary. It is typical for this vein to bulge like this when bleeding is indicated. Normally you should avoid bulging veins but in this case (11.26) it is okay to bleed slightly bulging veins such as this. This patient had delayed healing of an operation on his index finger, which was swollen and painful. After bleeding this vein, the pain diminished to zero. *Full-color picture at www.chinesebloodletting.com.*

Bleeding Tung point 44.07 Bei Mian (Back Face)

For all practical purposes, 44.07 is the same as TCM point LI15. It is especially indicated for chronic fatigue syndrome, but also for aching and soreness of the legs.

For bleeding purposes, it is best to think of it as an area rather than a point. Palpate for a good tender point and wet cup if you find one, using the McKesson 17g safety lancets and a cup small enough to fit snugly.

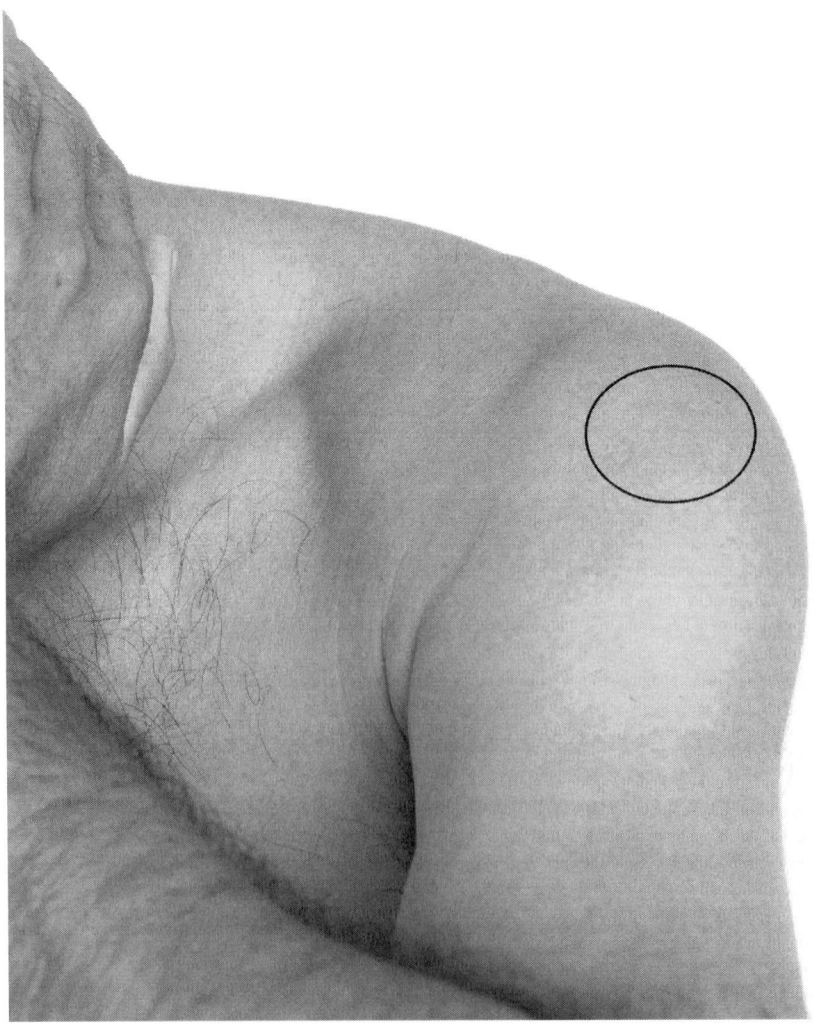

Fig. 10-9. 44.07 area

Additional areas to bleed

Bleeding Tung point 55.01 Huo Bao (Fire Bag)

This is the same point as the extra point *Du Yin*, and is located on the plantar side of the second toe, in the middle of the distal crease.

Master Tung bled this point for angina pectoris. In today's world, I would not treat a cardiac patient unless they were under the care of a physician.

This point is also bled for difficult labor (to help it along), retention of placenta, and liver conditions. Retention of placenta is treated medically these days; however, in the case of an incomplete miscarriage, 55.01 can be bled in an attempt to avoid surgical procedures such as a D&C.

These days, many women at the end of their pregnancy come in for "acupuncture inductions" to avoid having medical induction of labor. My own experience is that if the body is not ready, acupuncture cannot really "induce" labor. If the body *is* ready, acupuncture can help nudge the process along.

Bleeding point 55.01 can be an important part of treatment to prepare a woman for birth. Simply lance the point with a lancet or hypodermic needle. My preferred lancet for this is the McKesson 17g safety lancet. It will not be possible to cup there—simply lance and squeeze out some blood. Feet can harbor much pathogenic bacteria, so be sure to clean the area thoroughly beforehand, and cover with a sterile bandage afterwards.

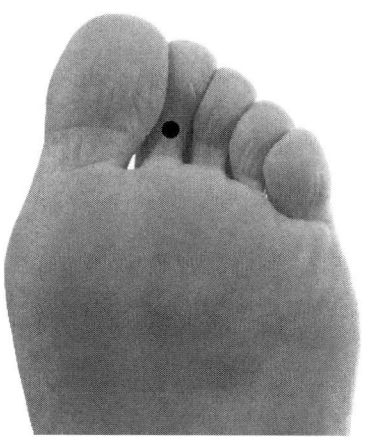

Fig. 10-10. 55.01

Bleeding Tung points 77.15 Shang Chun (Upper Lip and 77.16 Xia Chun (Lower Lip)

77.15 is located at the inferior edge of the patella, at the attachment to the patellar tendon. 77.16 is one cun below that.

While almost all bleeding on the legs is bleeding veins directly with no cupping necessary, these points are an exception—they are wet-cupped like points on the back.

These points are bled for lesions and sores, such as herpes on the lips of the mouth and genital area. 77.15 is also named Shang Chun (Upper Lip), and 77.16 is named Xia Chun (Lower Lip), for those are the areas they treat.

The best way to position a patient to bleed these points is to have them lie on their back with knees fully flexed. It is comfortable and convenient to have the patient put their feet apart, but place the knees together.[18]

Palpate at and around the points to find the most tender point, or simply bleed per textbook location. These are wet-cupped the same as points on the back, except that a smaller cup is called for.

If you do not have cups of the diameter necessary, you can simply squeeze out a little blood, which should work fine.

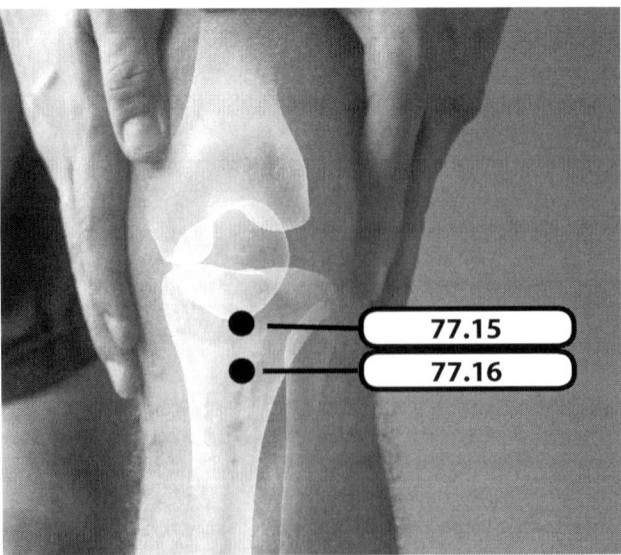

Fig. 10-11. 77.15 and 77.16

Bleeding the inside of the cheek

The go-to bleeding area for Bell's palsy in the Tung bleeding system is the oral mucosa—the inside of the cheek. It can be hard to see inside the mouth, so good lighting is helpful. If you don't have an assistant who can shine a flashlight, you can wear a "headlight," which allows you to clearly illuminate the inside of the mouth.

You can bleed the inside of the cheek with McKesson 17g safety lancets. Sometimes you will see a blue vein; best results can be obtained by bleeding such veins. If they are present you will be able to bleed them with better precision by using a hypodermic needle, 18g or 20g. If no such vein is present, just bleed 3-5 spots in the inside cheek superficially.

Some patients dislike the taste of their own blood, and find the idea of bleeding in their mouths unpleasant. So before doing this treatment, make sure the patient understands what will happen and is okay with it. Some patients have the attitude "sure, fine, whatever will help, let's do it." But if your patient seems unsure or hesitant after you explain the treatment, it is probably better to do something else.

I have also had good results bleeding the yang jing well points on the ipsilateral hand of Bell's palsy patients, which is readily accepted.

Bleeding for gout

Generally speaking, distal bleeding is more effective than local bleeding. Gout is an exception—it is best to wet-cup right where it is.

Gout is extremely painful, so generally it would be too excruciating to bleed right at the most painful point. So get as close as you can without it being too painful, and wet-cup as you would the back, using McKesson 17g safety lancets and a disposable cup.

The most common place for gout is the foot. Usually a large cup of the size used for cupping the back is too big, so you will need to use a smaller-size cup. You may not get a lot of blood but that's okay, whatever you get should alleviate the pain significantly.

Gout most often affects the joint at the base of the big toe (the MTP joint), but can also occur at other joints such as ankles, knees, wrists, fingers and elbows. Local wet-cupping is effective for gout no matter where the location.

When bleeding feet, keep in mind that they tend to harbor more pathogenic bacteria than other parts of the body. I usually swab first thoroughly with iodine (povidone iodine, or Betadine), then with alcohol. Always ask the patient if they are allergic to iodine. An alternative strong disinfectant is chlorhexidine gluconate.

Procedure for bleeding for gout

Bleeding for gout is wet-cupping, so the equipment and procedures are similar to wet-cupping the back as outlined in chapter 7. Use single-use disposable safety lancets, the smaller the gauge (the larger the diameter of the lancet) the better. I prefer the 17g McKesson disposable safety lancets (sold under the name "Acti-Lance" outside North America).

Gout often occurs in areas where a 50cm (2") cup will be too big. Determine where you will be cupping, then have a cup available of a size that will work there. It's a good idea to have a few cups of different sizes available so you can adjust the size if need be. Test to see if you can get a good air seal with the cup(s) you have available.

Gout most often occurs on the foot, especially in the metatarsophalangeal joint of the big toe. This area can harbor a lot of pathogenic bacteria and fungus, so I generally swab with both alcohol and a stronger disinfectant such as povidone iodine (Betadine).

Prepare your clean field with a few safety lancets, a few cotton balls or gauze, clean cups of sizes appropriate for the area to be bled, pump for cup inside of plastic bag, bandages and packaged alcohol wipes and/or stronger disinfectant such as povidone iodine (Betadine). Before using iodine, always ask the patient if he or she is allergic to it and if so, do not use.

Put on gloves. Clean the area you are about to bleed with an alcohol swab or other disinfectant. Take a safety lancet and twist the plastic stopper ¼ turn to remove and ready for use. With your thumb, palpate the area where the gout is. Gout is EXTREMELY painful so you probably cannot lance directly on the most tender spot as it will be too much. Using your judgment and communicating with your patient, find a spot as close to the most painful point as tolerable.

Place your safety lancet on that spot, press the button and discard. Depending on the area, use 2 or 3 lancets. Keep in mind that the punctures should be sufficiently close together that they will fit within the diameter of the cup you will be using.

Place the cup over the punctures and pump out air. The amount of blood you get will vary widely from patient to patient. You should get enough blood that some runs down and gathers at the inside rim of the cup. If that doesn't happen, you can remove the cup and swab the puncture area with alcohol, which thins the blood and encourages flow.

When you have enough blood, remove the cup carefully to avoid spillage. Discard the blood according to local regulations, along with any blood-tinged paper towels and cotton, and the cup. Remove the pump from the plastic bag, which should also be discarded.

Bleeding for shingles

For a patient with active shingles lesions, there is perhaps no more effective treatment in all of medicine than wet-cupping the lesions directly. It is best to do this while the lesions are fresh and active. Once they have healed over and the patient is suffering from post-herpetic neuralgia, treating it successfully is much more difficult.

For treating an active case of shingles, my preferred method is wet-cupping. Lance with McKesson/Acti-Lance 17g safety lancets and cup with disposable plastic cups.

The difference between this and most other wet-cupping is that you will use a LOT of safety lancets—4 or 5 for each lesion you cup. Determine approximately how many you will need and lay them out on your clean field in advance, as you do not want to be reaching into a box of safety lancets with gloved hands that have been in contact with blood and/or herpes-virus-laden fluid.

Also, take out in advance a disposable cup for each lesion you plan to cup, as each cup should be filled just once then thrown away. Why is this necessary? Because when the cup fills with blood or fluid and you remove it, the cup will be upside-down and the blood/fluid will gather at the valve. Some of it will remain near the valve even after you dispose of the liquid. If you use the cup again, when you pump, you may pull some droplets of infected fluid into your pump, putting future patients at risk of exposure.

Wet-cup each prominent lesion by making 3 to 5 punctures in each one, then cup.

You are dealing with fluids infected with the highly contagious herpes zoster virus, so extra caution is warranted. It is important to use eye protection—I always wear goggles when treating active shingles lesions. It is also a good idea to wear protective clothing that you can dispose of when you are done.

In China, practitioners often use plum blossom hammers on active shingles lesions, after which they may or may not cup. This method is thorough, simple, and effective, but it is painful for the patient and I would be concerned about "splattering" of herpes-laden fluids.

When you have finished, it is a good idea to dress the lesions to protect against infection. It may be too painful to place any adhesive near the lesions, so you can make large adhesive pads by cutting strips from 4" rolls and taping them together. That way you can place tape at the edge of the pads, far from the lesions. You can also buy pre-cut 9" x 5" sterile gauze pads.

WARNING!!! You can catch chickenpox from someone with shingles through contact with their secretions or rash—and possibly through airborne transmission if fluids from the rash become airborne. DO NOT treat shingles lesions directly or be in the vicinity of where it is being done if you are not certain you have immunity from chickenpox.

A note about bleeding Tai yang

A famous classical point to bleed is Tai yang, located at the temple, in the depression approximately one cun posterior to the midpoint between the lateral extremity of the eyebrow and the outer canthus of the eye. According to classical texts, this is bled for a wide variety of conditions including schizophrenia, mania, hypertension, diseases of the eyes and ears, headaches, toothaches, dizziness, trigeminal neuralgia and many more.

However, this is a difficult point to bleed. The visible vein should be bled, but often there is no visible vein or it is difficult to find. To make it stand out, some texts recommend having the patient (not the practitioner!!!) tighten the collar around their neck, while other sources warn this is a dangerous practice that could lead to stroke. There are arteries nearby that must be avoided. There is also a good possibility of bruising in this very visible spot.

For all these reasons, bleeding Tai yang is best avoided without specific training. The good news is that bleeding the apex of the ear is an excellent substitute for bleeding Tai yang. My experience is that bleeding the ear apex is just as effective as bleeding Tai yang in almost every case.

Chapter 11

Clinical guide to bloodletting by indication

To bleed or not to bleed?

Before we discuss *where* to bleed, let's first see how to determine whether or not it's even appropriate to bleed.

Some classic TCM signs of blood stasis are:

- Purple tongue
- Choppy pulse
- Engorged veins under tongue
- Purple lips and nails
- Bleeding with clots
- Fixed masses

Evaluating a patient for these signs of blood stasis can certainly help establish an overall clinical picture. To be perfectly honest, however, they are low on my list of criteria for determining whether or not to bleed.

Most patients come to me for help with specific, acute complaints. So my first consideration is not "Does this patient have signs of blood stasis?" Rather, the most relevant and direct question I can ask myself is: "Will bloodletting help resolve THIS COMPLAINT in THIS PATIENT?"

Following—in order of importance—are the considerations that in my experience can best help determine whether or not to bleed a specific patient for a specific complaint.

1. The nature of the complaint

Some complaints are best treated with bloodletting, period. If a patient comes in complaining of nausea for example, I always bleed DT.03 as this is the easiest, quickest, most painless and most effective treatment—a no-brainer.

Following—in no particular order—are some additional complaints that almost always call for bloodletting, and where to bleed:

- Gout (local bleeding)
- Trigeminal neuralgia (ipsilateral ear apex)
- Acute abdominal pain from any source (providing a physician has determined that emergency medical attention is not necessary) (veins on legs and/or ashi points in appropriate zones on back)
- High blood pressure (veins on legs or ear apex)
- Varicose veins (veins on ipsilateral leg—not the varicose veins themselves)
- Hemorrhoids (UB40 area)
- Shingles (local wet-cupping)
- Eye problems such as conjunctivitis, ptosis, optic neuritis, and more (ipsilateral ear apex)
- Radiating nerve pain or a pinched nerve, such as sciatica or numbness/tingling in the extremities

2. Palpation

Palpating for ashi points is appropriate when evaluating the back, buttocks or hips for bleeding (wet-cupping), and also for evaluating the VT areas on the front of the trunk. Generally speaking, however, palpation will not help evaluate legs, arms, ears, or other parts of the body for bleeding. (When bleeding legs or arms your eyes are your guide—you are looking for veins).

When a patient comes in with knee pain for example—particularly knee pain of a degenerative nature (for which the upper back area DT.07 is the premier zone to bleed)—the first thing I have them do is lie face down. Palpating that DT.07 zone in their upper back will determine how best to proceed.

The ideal finding would be one point in the DT.07 zone that is MUCH more tender to palpation than all the surrounding area—ideally a point so tender it makes the patient flinch, jump, or exclaim in pain. Finding such a point virtually guarantees that wet-cupping will treat the knee pain effectively. If you cannot find such a point, then do not bother bleeding the back as it will not work.

3. Patient history of having been successfully bled

If a particular patient has ever been successfully bled for ANY complaint, that patient is a "blood stasis type" and will generally respond to bloodletting. For these patients, bloodletting jumps to the top of the list of candidate therapies.

4. Presence of "bleedable-looking" veins

If a patient has dark, prominent, or easily-visible veins—particularly in the legs—this is suggestive of blood stasis and points in the direction of bloodletting.

5. Having exhausted other options

If you have tried the usual approaches to treating a particular problem and they have all failed, that in itself is sufficient reason to try bloodletting.

Headaches

If a patient comes in with a headache, there are two things I will do before doing acupuncture. First, I will dry cup their upper back on the side with symptoms, or both sides if the symptoms are bilateral. Often the headache is caused by tight muscles of the upper back, and cupping will help immediately. I only leave cups on for a minute or two at most, so this is quick.

Second, I will bleed the patient's ear apex on the same side as the headache, or both ears if the pain is bilateral. If the bleeding brings about some improvement, I will do additional bleeding (see below), either at that appointment or at their next appointment.

I prefer to see a patient while they are having a headache because if bleeding is going to work, the patient should notice a difference immediately. If they do respond immediately, I have a vitally important piece of information about this patient that will inform future treatments for headaches and anything else that patient may present with—I know this patient is in all probability a "blood-stasis type" with a blood-stasis-prone constitution. Whatever this patient presents with in the future, I now know that they are likely to respond to bloodletting.

Always be sure to get a baseline before bleeding so the patient is paying attention to the pain and can tell you if there's a change.

An area to bleed for headaches that is often even more powerful than bleeding the ear is the leg. The UB40 area is the most common area to bleed for this—it is the Master Tung occipital region. Also look for bleedable veins elsewhere on the legs, especially lateral lower legs.

The classic area to bleed for headaches is Tai yang but as mentioned, I generally substitute bleeding the ear for this, with excellent results.

Frontal headache

- Apex of the ear
- Visible veins on the leg, especially GB34/ST36 general area
- Frontal region of the feet (see page 121). Palpate and if you find a few particularly tender points, you can wet-cup them

Vertex headache

- Apex of the ear
- Visible veins on the leg, especially GB34/ST36 general area
- Yin tang (you can bleed this with a safety lancet. If the patient wants to avoid having a cupping mark there, you can simply squeeze out a few drops of blood).

Parietal headache

- Apex of the ear
- Visible veins on the leg, especially GB34/ST36 general area
- Palpate along the paraspinals, about 1.5 cun lateral to the spine and at approximately L2, for a very tender point. Bleed if you find one.

Occipital headache

- Apex of the ear
- Visible veins on the leg, especially the Master Tung "occipital zone" or UB40 area.
- Palpate along the paraspinals, about 1.5 cun lateral to the spine and at approximately L2, for a very tender point. Bleed if you find one.

Headaches involving the neck

- Apex of the ear
- Visible veins on the leg, especially the Master Tung "occipital zone" or UB40 area.
- Visible veins in the cubital fossa

Bell's palsy

- Yang jing well points on ipsilateral hand
- Inside of the cheek

Bell's palsy can be a difficult condition to treat, especially if many months have passed since onset. I have, however, often gotten good results with bleeding the yang jing well points of the ipsilateral hand.

The classic area to bleed for this is the inside cheek on the affected side. This is not hard to do using the McKesson 17g safety lancets. However, my experience with American patients is that many do not like this treatment. They taste their own blood which they then either have to swallow or go to a sink and spit out, then rinse their mouths. Patient acceptance can be a problem.

As mentioned, I've had good results bleeding the yang jing well points, and no problem with patient acceptance of this. I do acupuncture at every appointment as well.

Eye conditions

Also please see "Eye problems" on page 210 in Chapter 12—My favorite conditions to treat with bloodletting.

Optic neuritis

- Apex of the ear

There is little that Western medicine can do for patients with optic neuritis other than prescribe steroids, with limited effectiveness.

Bleeding the ear is far more effective. With a $.04 diabetic lancet and a simple poke or two, you can do more for optic neuritis patients than the most highly-trained physician using the most expensive medical equipment.

Temporal arteritis

- Apex of the ear

Like optic neuritis, the primary medical treatment for temporal arteritis causing vision loss is steroids. I have personally treated just one patient with this diagnosis, and the only treatment I used was bleeding the apex of his ear.

One patient treated is, of course, a small sample on which to base a claim of effectiveness. The patient responded well however, and felt that he regained a substantial amount of vision immediately following treatment.

Stye

- Apex of the ear
- GB14

Ptosis

- Apex of the ear

Bleeding the apex of the ear offers an effective alternative to surgery for patients with ptosis. It is not, however, a permanent fix—patients will need to repeat the treatment at regular intervals.

Conjunctivitis

- Apex of the ear
- UB 2
- LU 11

Keratitis

- Apex of the ear

Trigeminal neuralgia

- Apex of the ear and as described below

Trigeminal neuralgia (TN) is a terribly painful condition for which Western medicine has little to offer. By contrast, I am always happy to treat patients with trigeminal neuralgia, as they generally respond extremely well to simply bleeding their ipsilateral ear.

In the case of TN, I bleed the ear more thoroughly than just the apex—I also bleed a few more points along the helix, i.e. 99.08-1 and 99.08-2 as shown in Fig. 11-1 below. I may also bleed the tiny blue venule behind their ear—99.07—if I see one there.

The Complete Guide to Chinese Medicine Bloodletting

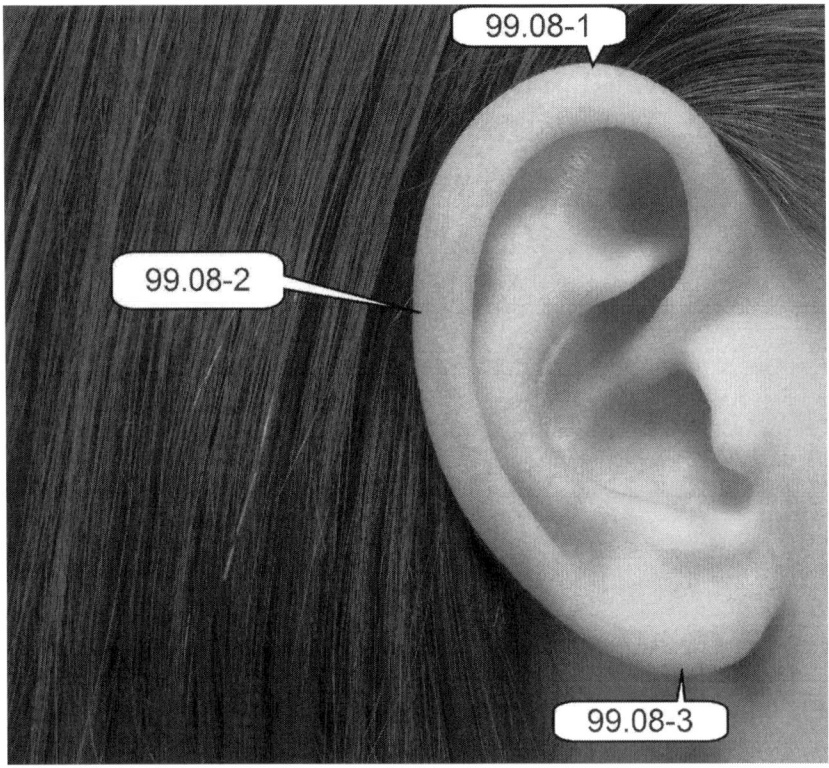

Fig. 11-1.

You can usually enhance effectiveness by bleeding the leg for this. The pain of TN is often confused with dental pain as it is in the same area. The Tung mouth/tooth region (see page 119) is on the lateral knee area, and that is first place to look for bleedable veins when treating TN.

However, you may find darker and more prominent veins elsewhere on that leg. As always, let your eyes be your guide—the "quality" of the veins is more important in determining where to bleed than where they are located.

Please see "Fay's trigeminal neuralgia" on page 217 in Chapter 13—Case studies. Also please see the entry "Trigeminal neuralgia" on page 177 in Chapter 12—My favorite conditions to treat with bloodletting.

Ear conditions

- Apex of the ear
- Visible veins on the leg, especially the Master Tung ear region (see page 119).

As a general rule, ear conditions can be treated by bleeding as indicated above

Otitis media

- Visible veins on the leg especially around the ankle
- 11.26

Nose conditions

Chronic sinusitis

- Apex of the ear
- Yin tang
- Master Tung frontal region of the foot (see page 121)

Rosacea

- 1010.12 (DU 25, the tip of the nose)
- Wet-cup UB20 and UB21

The tip of the nose can be easily bled with a safety lancet. No need to cup.

Nosebleed

- Wet-cup UB18

For nosebleeds in children, I have seen wet-cupping UB18 work a miracle. Wet-cup the tender point at or near UB18 on the side of the nosebleed. Two McKesson 17g safety lancets should suffice. Use a cup size appropriate for the size of the child.

Mouth conditions

Soreness and swelling of mouth, tongue, throat

- Apex of the ear
- Visible veins on the leg, especially the Master Tung mouth/tooth region (lateral to the knees, see page 119)
- LU 11 for soreness and swelling of the throat

Soreness and swelling of the lips

- 77.15 and 77.16

Toothache

- Apex of the ear
- Visible veins on the leg, especially the Master Tung mouth/tooth region (see page 119)

Jaw pain/TMJ and difficulty opening the mouth

- Apex of the ear
- Visible veins on the leg, especially the Master Tung mouth/tooth region (see page 119)

Neck conditions

Benign thyroid tumors, goiter

- VT.01
- Apex of the ear

Goiters can occur even in developed countries, although more often from Hashimoto's thyroiditis than from iodine deficiency. These can cause a variety of symptoms locally including difficulty swallowing, difficulty breathing, and a vague feeling of tightness or discomfort in the throat and surrounding area. Such symptoms can result from benign tumors of the thyroid gland as well.

Goiters and thyroid tumors should of course be medically managed by a physician. Acupuncture and particularly bloodletting can, however, significantly alleviate physical symptoms such as tightness and discomfort.

Bleeding the ear can be effective and offer the patient immediate relief. Also, you can bleed Master Tung point VT.01 for this. VT.01 is called a "nine-point unit," but it is really an area on the anterior neck. The main point is right at the Adam's apple, and you can bleed there. Pinch up the skin so that the needle is not going directly into the underlying structure, but rather just into the pinched-up skin, and use a McKesson 17g safety lancet or 21g manual lancet. You won't be able to cup there, just squeeze out a little blood.

Neck pain and stiffness

- Apex of the ear
- Visible veins in the leg, especially ST36/GB34 area and UB40 area
- Visible veins in the cubital fossa

Throat conditions

Tonsillitis, pharyngitis

- Apex of the ear
- LU11, LI1
- Visible veins in the cubital fossa
- Visible veins on the leg, especially ST 36/GB 34 region and UB40 region
- VT.01

Esophageal pain

- Apex of the ear
- Visible veins in the cubital fossa

- Visible veins on the leg, especially ST 36/GB 34 region and UB40 region
- VT.03

Upper limb conditions

In the Master Tung tradition, the most important area to bleed for issues of the upper limbs is the veins in the crook of the elbow. In a sense, this is the upper limb equivalent of bleeding UB40.

In my practice, however, the first place I bleed for upper limb issues is the apex of the ear, as this is so much easier than bleeding the crook of the elbow. For one thing, it requires less setup. Also, while it can be difficult to find good veins in the crook of the elbow, you never have a problem locating the apex of the patient's ear! And finally, it is easier to "sell" to the patient, as the patient doesn't see what you are doing and there is no risk of leaving a visible bruise.

In short, bleeding the ear is "no big deal" compared with bleeding the crook of the elbow.

If bleeding the apex of the ear produces a noticeable result, that is a clear indication that this is a blood stasis issue and that further bleeding will be effective. Additional areas to consider for bleeding are the legs, the upper back and, as mentioned, the veins in the crook of the elbow. See " What we can learn from phlebotomy about safely bleeding the cubital fossa" on page 152.

Shoulder and arm pain and numbness

- Apex of the ear
- Visible veins in the cubital fossa
- Visible veins on the leg, especially lower part of lateral leg
- Upper limb area of the back, general area of SI 10
- DT 16

Wrist pain

- Apex of the ear
- Visible veins in the cubital fossa

- Visible veins on the leg, especially lower part of lateral leg
- Upper limb area of the back, general area of SI 10

Hand and finger pain and numbness

- Apex of the ear
- Visible veins in the cubital fossa
- Visible veins on the leg, especially lower part of lateral leg
- Upper limb area of the back, general area of SI 10

Lower limb conditions

For any pain or symptom of the lower limbs, first bleed any visible veins in the UB40 area.

Also examine the legs and thighs for any veins that look particularly "bleedable," i.e. dark, prominent veins, and bleed those.

Pain and swelling of legs

- Visible veins in the UB40 region
- Visible veins anywhere else on the leg and thigh
- DT.08/09 area

Pain and numbness radiating down the legs/sciatica

- Visible veins in the UB40 region
- Visible veins anywhere else on the leg and thigh
- DT.08-DT.09 region
- If there is just one extremely tender point on the ipsilateral buttock, bleed there

When a patient tells me they have low back pain, my first question is "does the pain go down your leg?" If the answer is no, it's just in the low back and does not extend to the buttock or leg, then this is often a patient that does not need to be bled. I will try other approaches first and keep bleeding "in my back pocket" for use later if nothing else works.

But if the patient says the pain goes down their buttock, thigh, or leg, and particularly if that pain is one-sided, then bleeding is the first option to consider. Have them lie prone and evaluate for possible bleeding by palpating the DT.08-DT.09 area as pictured in Fig. 11-1 below. Also examine the backs of their legs for bleedable veins, particularly in the UB40 area.

The areas on the upper back to be bled for pain and numbness in the lower limbs are DT.08 and DT.09. DT.08 is described as being a two-point group, each point 6 cun lateral to the spine, one each lateral to the 2nd and 3rd thoracic vertebrae. DT.09 is described as being a group of three points, also 6 cun lateral to the spine, at the level of the 4th, 5th, and 6th thoracic vertebrae.

In practice however, it is best to think of these two "groups" as a single area to be bled, as in the illustration below. Essentially, this is the area at and near the medial border of the scapula.

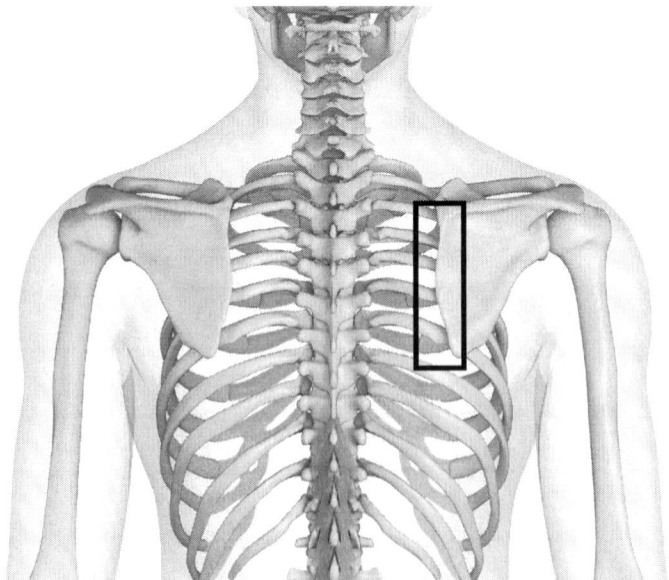

Fig. 11-2. Tung DT.08-DT.09 area

To bleed, have the patient lie prone and palpate that area. Again, you are looking for a point that is markedly more tender to palpation than the surrounding area. The more tender it is, the better. If the patient reacts strongly by flinching or gasping when you press, bleeding that point is virtually certain to be successful.

Assuming you find that tender point, you can further verify its validity by palpating the mirror point on the contralateral side. So for example if the patient has symptoms on the right side, and their right UB43 is tender to palpation, palpate the left UB43. If it is NOT tender, that is further confirmation that the tenderness of right UB43 correlates to the leg pain, and that bleeding that point will be successful.

If you cannot find any points that are tender despite your best efforts, then you can forget about bleeding the back of this patient. It will not work.

The second area to bleed for sciatica and sciatica-like pain is the UB40 area. This does NOT mean the acupuncture point UB40, but a broad area on the back of the legs and the sides of the legs roughly centered at UB40. This is the Master Tung "occipital region" as shown on page 120.

Where exactly to bleed? Remember that bleeding legs is different from bleeding the back. On the back there are generally no veins to see, so palpation is your guide. But when bleeding legs you are bleeding veins, so your eyes will tell you where. You are looking for bleedable veins. See " A gallery of veins to bleed and veins to avoid" on page 122.

Please also see "Rebecca's sciatica" on page 225 and "Dale's left sciatica and knee" on page 233 in Chapter 13—Case studies. Also please see the entry "Sciatica" on page 206 in Chapter 12—My favorite conditions to treat with bloodletting.

Knee pain

- DT.07
- Bleeding veins on the legs locally (not often indicated but occasionally)

In all of Chinese medicine, I don't believe there is a more "magical" treatment than bleeding the famous Master Tung point DT.07 for knee pain, particularly knee pain caused by a degenerative condition.

DT.07 is typically described as 3 points, 3 cun lateral to the thoracic spine, lateral to the 3rd, 4th and 5th intercostal spaces. But that would put the points at the medial border of the scapula, and in reality they are most commonly found between the medial border of the scapula and spine, as pictured in Fig. 11-3 below.

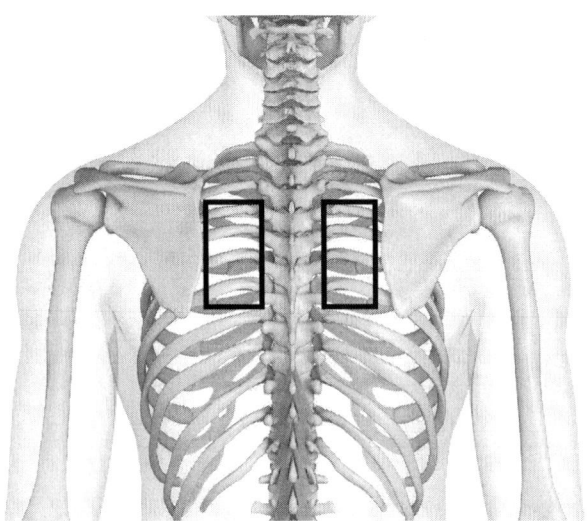

Fig. 11-3. DT.07 for knee pain.

Evaluating the patient to see if this treatment will be effective is simple—just have the patient lie prone and palpate that area on the upper back, ipsilateral to the pain. You are looking for a point that is markedly more tender to palpation than the surrounding area. The more tender it is, the better. If the patient reacts strongly by flinching or gasping when you press there, then bleeding that point is virtually certain to be successful.

Assuming you find that tender point, you can further verify its validity by palpating the mirror point on the contralateral side (providing the contralateral knee is not painful as well).

So for example, if the patient has right knee pain and you find a point within the right DT.07 area that is tender to palpation, palpate their left side at the same, mirror-image point. If it is NOT tender, that is further confirmation that the tenderness of the right point you found correlates to the knee pain, and that bleeding it will be successful.

If you cannot find any points that are tender despite your best efforts, then forget about bleeding this point on this patient; it will not work.

When the patient comes back for their next appointment, say, a few days or a week later, you will still be able to see where you bled. Palpate around that area and you will find a new "most-tender" spot. Bleed there—that will give your patient additional relief.

On rare occasions, bleeding locally is what's needed. If the patient has no point tender to palpation in the DT.07 area, and particularly if the knee pain is the result of an injury rather than a degenerative process, try bleeding veins locally in the ipsilateral leg.

Please see "Delia's knee" on page 235, and "Dale's left sciatica and knee" on page 233 in Chapter 13—Case studies. Also please see the entry "Knee pain" on page 205 in Chapter 12—My favorite conditions to treat with bloodletting.

Ankle pain

- Visible veins on the leg, especially the UB40 region, ST36/GB34 region, and around the ankle

Foot pain and numbness

- Visible veins in the UB40 region
- Visible veins around the ankle
- Visible veins anywhere else on the leg and thigh

If the pain is the result of pain radiating down the legs from the buttock region, see "Pain radiating down the legs/sciatica" above.

Heel pain/plantar fasciitis

- Visible veins in the UB40 region
- Visible veins around the ankle
- Visible veins anywhere else on the leg and thigh

You can classify plantar fasciitis/heel pain into two categories—the ones that don't respond at all to bloodletting, and those that respond dramatically. There doesn't seem to be a middle ground.

How to know which is which? No obvious way, you just have to bleed and see. Where? UB40 is the go-to, but as always when bleeding veins on the legs, bleed what you see. If you see bleedable veins somewhere other than UB40, bleed those too.

Longstanding foot pain that will not heal

- 11.26 "Control dirt"
- Visible veins in the UB40 region

- Visible veins around the ankle
- Visible veins anywhere else on the leg and thigh

Two of my most amazing success stories with bleeding were women with foot pain that had lasted more than a year despite extensive medical interventions. Both were due to fractures that would not heal, i.e. non-union of bone. Please see "Katie's 3-year foot ordeal" on page 215 and "Sheila's heel that wouldn't heal" on page 216 in Chapter 13—Case studies.

Both cases resolved quickly after bleeding 11.26.

Hip pain

- Wet-cup locally

There is no Master Tung bleeding zone on the back or legs for hip pain. However, I have often had success bleeding (wet-cupping) locally at or near the greater trochanter.

This is the same procedure as wet-cupping the back. Have the patient side-lying, with the painful hip facing up. Palpate the area, especially on and around the greater trochanter. The best finding in terms of probable success would be to find a single point that is the focus of the pain on palpation—a point significantly more tender to palpation than the surrounding area.

The patient will not be aware that there is a single focal point of pain on palpation waiting to be found—usually they will report that the whole area is tender to palpation. You will have to be a good and persistent "detective" to find that one tender point that is significantly *more* tender. But in most cases it is there, waiting to be found.

Wet-cupping the hip at or near the greater trochanter yields very little blood, literally a tiny drop at each of the punctures. Still, it can often significantly relieve pain.

Chest conditions

Pain in the chest area

- Apex of the ear
- Visible veins in the leg, especially lateral leg

- Visible veins in the UB40 region
- Visible veins anywhere else on the leg and thigh

Asthma/difficulty breathing

- Lung area of the back as shown Fig. 11-4 below. Palpate for tender points and wet-cup there. Usually 2 cups each side.
- Cubital fossa
- Visible veins in the leg, especially lateral leg (Master Tung lung region)

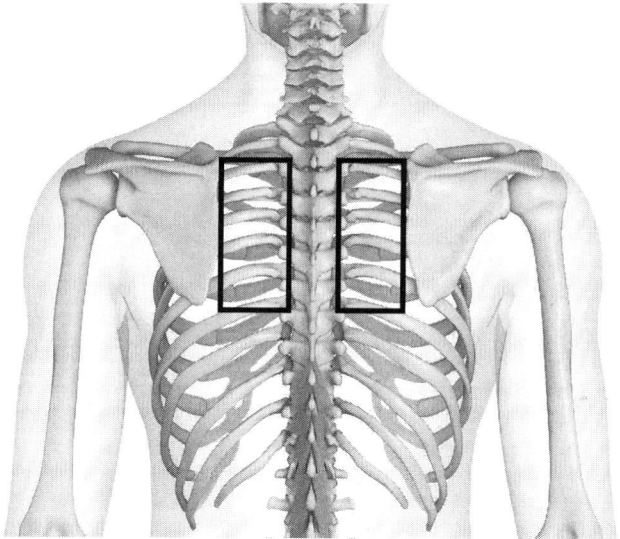

Fig. 11-4. Lung zone

Bronchitis

- Lung area of the back as shown above. Palpate for tender points and wet-cup there. Usually 2 cups each side.
- Cubital fossa
- Visible veins in the leg, especially lateral leg (Master Tung lung region)

Cardiac conditions

- Visible veins in the left cubital fossa

- DT.11, particularly to the left of the spine. Palpate and wet-cup where tender
- Visible veins on the lateral left leg

Angina pectoris

- Visible veins on the lateral left leg
- Visible veins in the left cubital fossa
- DT.11, particularly to the left of the spine. Palpate and wet-cup where tender
- 55.01

Abdominal conditions

I have had extraordinary success bleeding for all kinds of abdominal pain, including difficult and painful conditions such as interstitial cystitis, inflammatory bowel syndrome, inflamed kidney, endometriosis and more. I have also found bleeding highly effective for reflux. And in at least one case of severe non-stop nerve pain in the abdomen caused by nerve entrapment following surgery, bleeding resulted in dramatic, long-term relief.

In almost every case of abdominal pain, bleeding will give results far superior to filiform needling.

The best place to bleed for most cases of abdominal pain is the legs. Remember that means you are looking for *veins* in the leg—for more details, refer to Chapter 8—Bleeding legs. The most likely areas to find suitable veins to bleed are the lateral lower leg (ST36 region, broadly speaking) and the UB40 area.

Please see the entry "Abdominal pain, including cramps, endometriosis, interstitial cystitis and more" on page 207 in Chapter 12—My favorite conditions to treat with bloodletting.

Interstitial cystitis

- Visible veins in the legs, especially the ST36/GB34 area
- Visible veins in the UB40 region

Interstitial cystitis is a stubbornly painful condition for which Western medicine has no good treatment. Those who have it—mostly women—suffer terribly.

Bleeding can offer great—and often instantaneous—relief. Best points are usually found in the lateral lower leg (ST36 area) and UB40 area. I don't believe you will find any treatment in Western or Chinese medicine that is as effective.

A good example is a 39-year-old elementary school teacher, Tasha. She had constant flareups of IC with pain in her lower abdomen that made it difficult to function. Her story is in Chapter 13—Case studies. See "Tasha's interstitial cystitis" on page 221

Post-surgical pain/pinched nerve

- Visible veins on the leg, especially the lateral leg
- Visible veins in the UB40 region
- Local points tender to palpation

See "Deborah's post-surgical entrapped nerve" on page 220 in Chapter 13—Case studies

Liver/Gall bladder conditions

- Visible veins on the lower leg, especially the GB 34 region
- Palpate the right back area from UB17 to UB23 and wet-cup any very tender points
- 55.01

Pain from gallstones

- Palpate the right bladder channel from approximately L2 to L5, and wet-cup any very tender points
- Visible veins in the lateral right leg

Hepatitis

- Visible veins on the lower leg, especially ST36 region
- Visible veins in the cubital fossa

- Palpate the right back area from UB17 to UB23 and wet-cup any very tender points

Gastric and digestive conditions and pain

- Visible veins on the lower leg, especially ST36 region, also UB40 region, and the Master Tung "stomach region" on the legs page 121.
- DT.15. Palpate and wet-cup where tender

See "Ben's severe abdominal cramps" on page 218 in Chapter 13—Case studies

Kidney conditions/nephritis

- VT.05 palpate for very tender point and wet-cup there, most likely the point above and to the left or right of the navel, depending on which side the pain is
- 44.17 (same as SI 10)
- Visible veins on the leg, especially the lateral leg
- Palpate the bladder channel from approximately L2 to S4 and bleed any points that are very tender to palpation

See "Maria's recurrent kidney infections" on page 231 in Chapter 13—Case studies

Clinical guide to bloodletting by indication

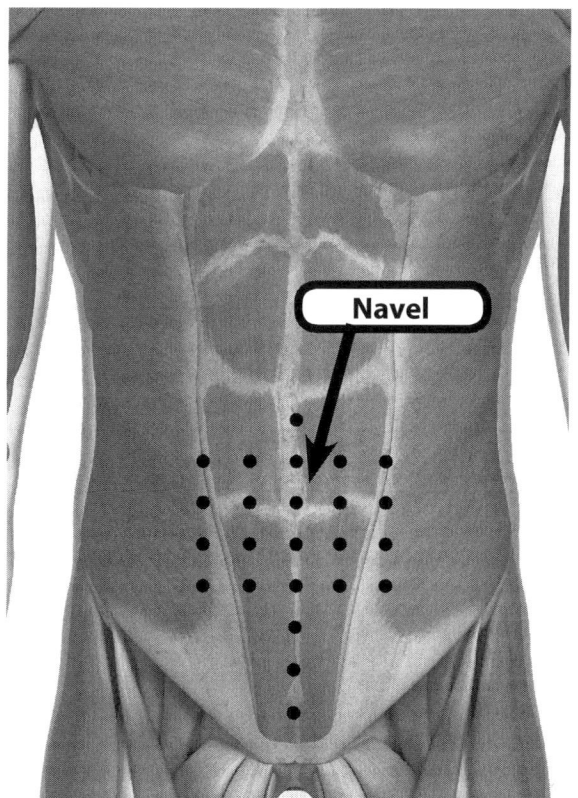

Fig. 11-5. VT.05

Pain from kidney stones

- VT.05 palpate for a very tender point and wet-cup there
- 44.17 (same as SI 10)
- Visible veins on the leg, especially the lateral leg

Back pain

Upper back pain

- Apex of the ear
- Palpate for the most tender point on the upper back and wet-cup it directly

- Visible veins in the leg, especially the UB40 region

Low back pain

- Visible veins on the legs, especially the UB40 region
- Palpate the low back and wet-cup any points that are very tender to palpation

Coccyx pain

- Visible veins in the leg (see "Samantha's coccyx pain" on page 212).

Spinal cord injury

- Palpate all along the paraspinals and wet-cup wherever tender. There may be several spots to bleed. Palpate gently at first as SCI patients may be VERY sensitive in that area7-27-18. See "Charles' spinal cord injury" on page 211.

Gynecological conditions

Amenorrhea

- DT.15

Dysmenorrhea

- DT.15
- Visible veins in the leg, especially the UB40 region and ST 36 region, also the area between the medial malleolus and SP 6

Endometriosis

- DT.15
- Visible veins in the leg, especially the UB40 region and ST 36 region, also the area between the medial malleolus and SP 6

Endometriosis is another condition that responds exceptionally well to bleeding. Best place to bleed is the legs, UB40 area or lateral lower legs—or wherever you find the best, most bleedable veins.

Please see "Margaret's endometriosis" on page 219 in Chapter 13—Case studies. Also please see "Abdominal pain, including cramps, endometriosis, interstitial cystitis and more" on page 207 in Chapter 12—My favorite conditions to treat with bloodletting.

Infertility

- Visible veins in the leg, especially the UB40 region and ST 36 region, also the area between the medial malleolus and SP 6

Mastitis

- Apex of the ear and helix posterior ear point
- Visible veins in the leg, especially the UB40 region and ST 36/GB 34 region

Uterine fibroids

- Visible veins in the leg, especially the UB40 region and ST 36 region, also the area between medial malleolus and SP 6

Circulatory system conditions

Stroke

- All jing well points, especially during the acute phase and in case of coma.

High blood pressure

- Apex of the ear
- Visible veins in the legs, especially lower medial and lateral legs near the ankles

Hypertension, or high blood pressure, is another indication for which bloodletting can often produce immediate, dramatic results.

Be aware that once a patient has high blood pressure, the act of taking their blood pressure can cause anxiety, making the blood pressure reading higher than it normally is. To overcome this, it is useful have patients buy an automatic, push-button blood pressure cuff, and bring it to the clinic. After treating them, have them lie down, put the cuff on their arm, and instruct them to take their blood pressure repeatedly, every few minutes.

Most often, by the end of the session their blood pressure is way down. You can tell them "this is what your blood pressure is when you're not thinking about your blood pressure," which is reassuring to them. They then have the confidence to not get so anxious at their doctor's office, and the reading there becomes more accurate as well.

Please see "Frank's high blood pressure" on page 222 in Chapter 13—Case studies. Also the entry "High blood pressure" on page 208 in Chapter 12—My favorite conditions to treat with bloodletting.

Varicose veins

- Do NOT bleed the ropey, bulging varicose veins themselves. Instead, bleed dark, flat veins on the same leg.

If I were to open a clinic dedicated to treating just one condition, it might well be varicose veins. Bloodletting makes them so easy to treat, the treatment is so effective, and patients are so happy, that treating them is a joy.

First, let's define our terms, as many people confuse varicose veins with spider veins.

Varicose veins are those ropey, green, protruding veins such as those in Figs. 11-6 and 11-7 below.

Clinical guide to bloodletting by indication

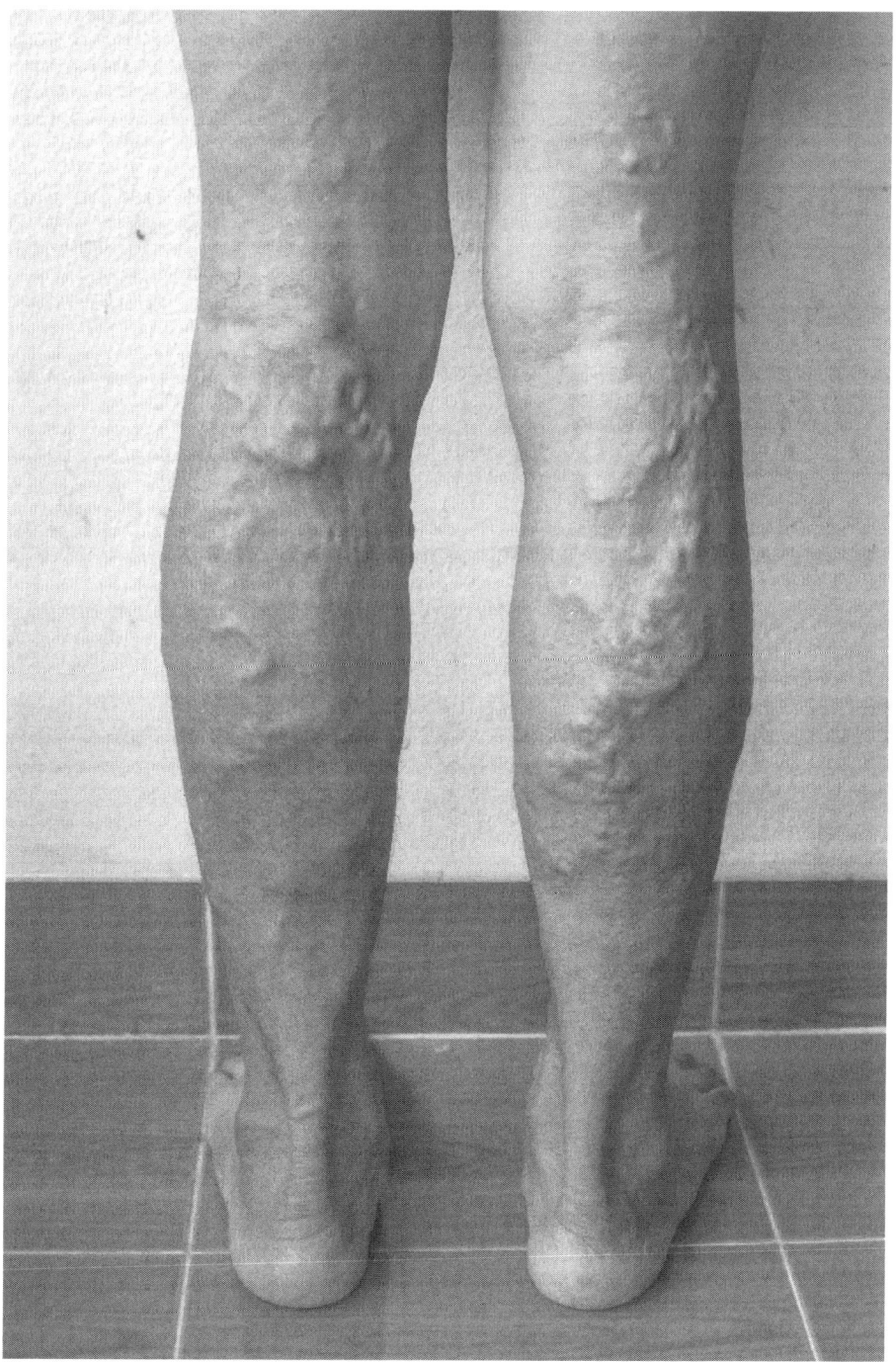

Fig. 11-6. Varicose veins

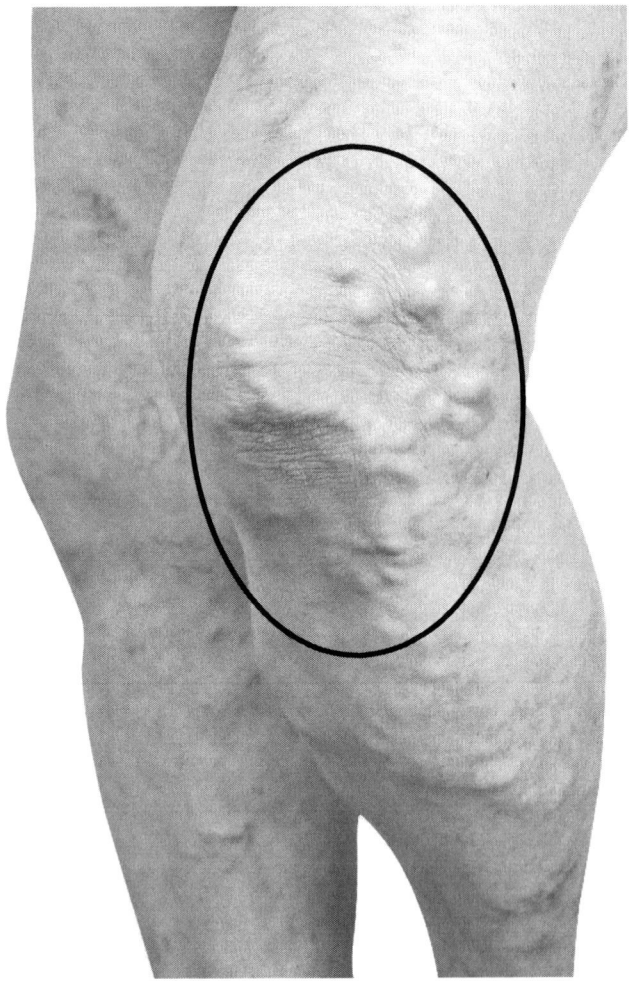

Fig. 11-7. Varicose veins (circled).

Do not bleed ropey, distended varicose veins such as these; doing so would only make them more distended.

However, on the same leg as the varicose veins, you will almost always find dark, prominent, flat veins. These are "spider veins." It is effective to bleed spider veins to treat varicose veins on the same leg.

You will find that when you bleed spider veins, varicose veins on that leg will shrink, sometimes immediately. Any pain caused by the varicose veins should also diminish significantly.

Please see "Matthew's varicose veins" on page 214, and "Helen's 'stealth' varicose vein treatment" on page 215 in Chapter 13—Case studies. Also please see the entry "Varicose veins" on page 208 in Chapter 12—My favorite conditions to treat with bloodletting.

Other conditions

Hemorrhoids

- UB40 area
- Visible veins in the leg, especially SP9 area and back of calf

For hemorrhoids, bloodletting is amazingly effective.

Hemorrhoids are essentially varicose veins of the anus and lower rectum and, like varicose veins, they respond exceptionally well to bloodletting. This alone will usually resolve even the worst cases of hemorrhoids. A few treatments may be necessary.

Please see "David's hemorrhoids" on page 218 in Chapter 13—Case studies. Also please see the entry "Hemorrhoids" on page 209 in Chapter 12—My favorite conditions to treat with bloodletting.

Skin conditions

- Apex of the ear
- Visible veins on the legs

Poison ivy/poison oak

- DT.01/DT.02 area
- Apex of the ear

Nausea and vomiting

- DT.03

If I had to choose my number one favorite indication to treat with bloodletting, it might well be nausea. This treatment is quick and easy, and also exceptionally effective.

For this I recommend McKesson 17g safety lancets. With the patient lying prone, pinch up the skin on the back of the neck just above the hairline, then prick twice and squeeze out a bit of blood. Cupping is not necessary, and would be difficult due to the hair.

I cannot recall a single time this treatment has failed to relieve nausea immediately.

Please see "Veronica's nausea" on page 230 in Chapter 13—Case studies. Also please see the entry "Nausea" on page 205 in Chapter 12—My favorite conditions to treat with bloodletting.

Depression, stress, insomnia, anxiety

- Apex of the ear

I bleed the ear apex of virtually every patient who presents for anxiety, depression, insomnia, severe stress or other emotional upset/psychological disturbance. Only one ear at a time needs to be bled. Depending on how severe the symptoms are, I may bleed an ear at every visit or just occasionally.

Some patients come in every week over an extended period of time for these symptoms. In that case I may alternate ears, bleeding the right ear one week and the left ear the next week. I also vary the location on the ear so that one week I will bleed the apex, next week a centimeter back from that, the next week further down, etc. That way I do not repeat bleeding the same spot until many weeks later. Doing it this way I can continue bleeding an ear every week indefinitely.

Many patients will feel an immediate "release" or lessening of symptoms. I usually begin the session by bleeding their ear, then needle.

By many accounts, bleeding is effective for schizophrenia. Two Chinese books written in the 1980's by Chinese bloodletting experts—Ci Xue Yi Jin (The Medical Mirror of Bloodletting) and Ci Xue Liao Fa (The Bleeding Book of Wang Xiuzhen) speak at length about treating schizophrenia with bloodletting.

It is not clear, however, exactly what they mean by "schizophrenia." One writes, for example, that bloodletting is most effective in schizophrenia caused by emotional trauma or major life changes, which sounds more like PTSD than schizophrenia as understood in western medicine. It really falls under the TCM classification of mania/madness.

In any case, the main bleeding points recommended by these authors are Tai yang, PC3 and UB40. As mentioned earlier, you can safely substitute bleeding the apex of the ear for bleeding Tai yang.

Chronic non-healing ulcers and injuries, and non-union of bones

- 11.26

Whenever a patient complains of a chronic non-healing wound, ulcer or bone that should have healed but has failed to do so, consider bleeding 11.26.

While I have not had occasion to bleed 11.26 often, I have had some spectacular results when I did. This includes two women with longstanding foot pain, one of whom had been on crutches for over a year. See "Katie's yearlong foot ordeal" on page 215 and "Sheila's heel that wouldn't heal" on page 216 in Chapter 13—Case studies.

Another patient, Paul, had unrelenting pain for many months following surgery on an arthritic finger. This too resolved shortly after bleeding 11.26.

Concussion

- KD 2

Gout

- Local wet-cupping as close to the center of the pain as possible.

In most cases, distal bleeding is more effective than local bleeding. Gout, however, is an exception—you wet-cup for gout right where it is.

Gout is extremely painful, so it would be too excruciating to bleed right at the most painful point. So get as close as you can without it being too painful, and wet-cup using the McKesson 17g safety lancets and a disposable cup.

The most common place for gout to occur is the foot. Usually a large cup of the size used for cupping the back is too big to fit snugly, so you will need to use a smaller-size cup. You may not get a lot of blood but that's okay, whatever you get should alleviate the pain significantly.

One more consideration with bleeding feet is that they tend to harbor more pathogenic bacteria than other parts of the body, so careful disinfection is recommended. I usually swab first thoroughly with iodine (povidone iodine, or Betadine), then with alcohol. Always ask the patient first if they are allergic to iodine.

Please see "Gout" on page 206 in Chapter 12—My favorite conditions to treat with bloodletting.

Fever

- Apex of the ear
- The 12 jing well points

Shingles

- Wet-cup directly on the lesions

Bleeding directly on the lesions is miraculously effective for shingles, and can often resolve the pain in one treatment. This is most effective when the lesions are still active—the earlier you treat it, the better.

Even if untreated, shingles lesions will generally resolve in a few weeks. Often, however, the severe pain does not go away but instead continues non-stop. This condition is called post-herpetic neuralgia, and the misery and suffering it can cause is difficult to describe. It can last anywhere from several weeks to decades—sometimes for the rest of a person's life.

Wet-cupping can help ease the pain of post-herpetic neuralgia, although this is much more difficult to treat at this stage than at the active-lesion stage. It can also be difficult for a patient to specify exactly where the pain is coming from once the active lesions are gone, although some scarring often remains, which can help guide where to cup.

Be aware that the lesions and fluid within them carry the herpes virus that causes shingles. Take extra precautions, keeping this in mind. It is crucial to immediately discard anything that the lesions or fluids touch. Wear goggles, and be particularly careful to avoid any "splattering" of fluid.

When wet-cupping active shingles lesions, I recommend using the 17g McKesson safety lancets and disposable plastic cups. Most cases of shingles occur on one side of the body, from the back around to the breast area. Have the patient lie on the non-affected side, exposing the front, back, and affected side, and wet-cup all the major lesions.

Be sure to set aside enough time—and enough safety lancets—to do a thorough job. If you do it thoroughly enough, you probably will not have to do it a second time. Alternatively, you could use manual diabetic lancets or hypodermic needles, although this would be more painful.

Some practitioners—particularly in China—prefer plum blossom hammers for this, but personally I would be concerned about the "splattering" of virus-laden fluid.

Before bleeding active lesions, make sure you have a plan how you will dress them once you are done. I recommend having on hand large sterile gauze pads (9" x 5" works well) or rolls of 4" sterile gauze you can cut to size. You can tape these together to make even larger pads if necessary so when you apply tape to affix the gauze to the skin, the tape will be far from the very sensitive lesions.

Please see "Shingles" on page 206 in Chapter 12—My favorite conditions to treat with bloodletting.

Bedwetting in children

- Wet-cup DU 2

Herpes and sores of the lips and genitals

- 77.15 and 77.16
- Apex of the ear (lesions on the lips of the mouth)

Chapter 12

My favorite conditions to treat with bloodletting

Following, in no particular order, are the indications that, in my experience, respond best to bloodletting.

Nausea

If I had to pick one indication to treat with bloodletting that combines the best features of effectiveness, quickness, and simplicity, it might well be nausea. This treatment is pure magic.

The Master Tung "point" DT.03 is bled for nausea. What that means in reality is that you have the patient lie prone, pinch up a bit of skin in the back of the neck, and prick once or twice just above the hairline (approximately ½" or 10mm above the hairline, precision is not important). I like to use 17g McKesson safety lancets for this. It's difficult to cup there due to the hair, so simply squeeze out a bit of blood.

The response is usually immediate, dramatic, and long-lasting. More information on page 199.

Knee pain

For knee pain—particularly if the pain is from a degenerative condition—no treatment is more effective than bleeding the Master Tung "point" or zone DT.07. That is true even in cases where the patient has failed cortisone injections, Synvisc injections, etc. More information on page 185.

Sciatica, especially when radiating down the UB channel

If a patient has low back pain in a fixed location, bleeding may or may not help. If the pain is radiating down their leg however, bleeding is always the treatment of choice. Details on page 183.

Gout

The pain of gout can be debilitating, and quick relief is hard to find. Western medicine has little to offer. A change of diet can help prevent future attacks but does nothing in the short term.

Bleeding locally, however, can offer immediate pain relief. Detailed instructions are on page 201.

Trigeminal neuralgia

Trigeminal neuralgia causes facial pain along the trigeminal nerve. While not life threatening, the pain can be unbearable.

Western medicine treatments include anticonvulsant drugs, botox injections, neurosurgery, and radiation therapy (gamma knife). These treatments carry considerable risk and rarely work well. In my experience, none of the western medical treatments match the effectiveness—and certainly the safety—of simply bleeding the apex of the ear.

In this case—just to be thorough as the condition is so debilitating—I bleed a few points along the helix of the ear from 99.08-1 to 99.08-2. Additional details on page 177.

My favorite conditions to treat with bloodletting

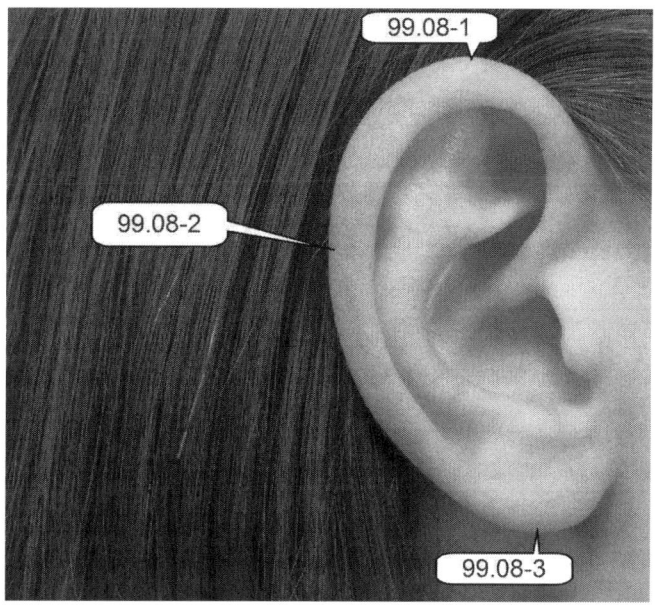

Fig. 12-1.

Abdominal pain, including cramps, endometriosis, interstitial cystitis and more

Severe abdominal pain should always be referred to a physician first to rule out serious pathology. Assuming that has been done, bloodletting is the intervention most likely to produce immediate, dramatic relief.

Bleeding can impact abdominal pain from a wide variety of causes. Whatever the source of the abdominal pain—be it stomach cramps, endometriosis, interstitial cystitis and more, your patient will generally get immediate relief if you bleed their legs. Look for visible veins in the UB40 area and the ST36/GB34 area (lateral upper leg).

Nothing else in Chinese Medicine—or perhaps any other medicine for that matter—can approach the power of bloodletting for severe abdominal pain.

High blood pressure

Nobody denies that high blood pressure can cause many potentially lethal conditions including kidney failure, heart disease, stroke, and more. But in a rational world, bloodletting—not drugs—would be the first line of therapy for it.

That is because the drugs used to combat hypertension are not benign. They can cause fatigue, dizziness, headaches, constipation, diarrhea, drowsiness, GERD, muscle and joint ache, and many more ill effects.

Bloodletting for hypertension can be as effective as drugs, and sometimes more so. Hypertension patients often have dark veins in their lower medial or lateral legs; if you find such veins, bleeding them will generally be highly effective. If the bleedable veins are elsewhere on the patient's legs, remember to "bleed what you see, wherever it may be."

Simply bleeding the apex of one or both ears can be highly effective as well.

Once a patient has high blood pressure, the act of taking their blood pressure becomes unpleasant and traumatic, as it is associated with bad news. The result is a vicious circle in which the mere act of taking the patient's blood pressure itself raises their blood pressure, making it difficult to determine what the blood pressure is when they're not thinking about it.

For that reason, I have patients buy an automatic blood pressure cuff—one for which they need only press a button, and the cuff inflates and does the rest. After bloodletting or at the next visit, I insert needles then have the patient lie down with the blood pressure cuff on their arm, and tell them to take and retake their blood pressure every few minutes. Over time they settle down and their blood pressure invariably drops. Usually by the end of the session the reading is much reduced, often in the normal range. More details on page 195.

Varicose veins

When my patient is happy, I'm happy. And no patients are happier than the ones I bleed for those ropey, bulging, unsightly varicose veins.

This treatment almost never fails to dramatically shrink varicose veins. Legs look much better after treatment. Even more important, patients feel better. Some patients have painful varicose veins that affect their sleep, and the pain is vastly reduced if not eliminated after treatment. Even patients who had not complained of pain often tell me their legs feel "lighter."

The benefits of this treatment are long-lasting as well. The patient may have to come back for a "tune-up" from time to time, but not often.

Never bleed the varicose veins themselves—find dark, flat veins on the same leg and bleed those. See page 196 for more details.

Hemorrhoids

Hemorrhoids are essentially varicose veins of the rectum. And like varicose veins, they can be successfully treated in most cases by bloodletting.

The main area to bleed for hemorrhoids is the UB40 area (also called the occipital zone in Master Tung bloodletting).

Hemorrhoid surgery is painful and carries a fairly high risk of complications, including bleeding, fissure, fistula, abscess, stenosis, urinary retention, soiling, incontinence and infection.

In many if not most cases, these painful, expensive and sometimes debilitating complications can be avoided by simply bleeding the UB40 area. More details on page 199.

Shingles

There is perhaps no pain worse than the pain of shingles, and mainstream medicine has little for it. The doctor can write a prescription for antiviral drugs but if they help, it is only marginally.

You, however, can virtually eliminate the pain of an active shingles outbreak by lancing the lesions and—if you wish—wet-cupping them. I like to cup after lancing for the sake of thoroughness. Some practitioners, however, lance or plum-blossom without cupping, and that works also.

If the active lesions are not lanced, then the patient faces the possibility of post-herpetic neuralgia. This is excruciating pain that continues well after the active lesions heal—sometimes for the rest of a person's life.

More details on page 202.

Eye problems

I have treated only a few cases of each of the following, but in virtually every case the patient got immediate relief from bleeding the ipsilateral ear apex.

- Temporal arteritis causing vision problems.
- Ptosis
- Conjunctivitis
- Stye
- Ocular neuritis

Chapter 13

Case studies

Charles' spinal cord injury

Charles is a 34 year old patient who suffered a spinal cord injury (SCI) during a motocross race 4 years ago. He has a scar from T8 to L3 and tells me that his spine was fused from T9 to T12 during an 8-hour surgery following the accident. His injury is the neurological equivalent of his spinal cord being severed at L1, and he is in a wheelchair.

Like most SCI patients, Charles suffers from severe chronic pain. He has tried to find relief with many therapies including chiropractic, Active Release Technique, physical therapy, massage, several acupuncturists, and more, with varying success. Charles' pain is mostly in his back.

At our first few appointments, I tried a variety of approaches including gua sha, cupping, scalp acupuncture and needling the HTJJ points directly with e-stim. Charles did get some relief but not as much as either of us had hoped for, so I decided to try bloodletting.

I found several areas tender to palpation along Charles' paraspinals, mostly to the right of the scar and especially toward the bottom, near L3. I prepared 4 disposable cups and 16 McKesson 17g safety lancets, and wet-cupped the four most tender areas along the spine.

A week later Charles came back and enthusiastically reported that the treatment had given him more relief than any he had done in the four years since his injury. He requested the same treatment again.

Charles has been in four more times since the initial bleeding treatment and each time asks for wet-cupping along the spine, as "this is really working." His wife also told him that his "guitar strings"—his very tight paraspinals—had softened considerably.

It is gratifying to be able to give Charles some relief from the constant debilitating pain. Sadly, the majority of SCI patients live with such pain. I hope that more acupuncturists will offer wet-cupping along the spine as an option to their SCI patients.

Samantha's coccyx pain

When Samantha told me she had pain in her coccyx, I groaned silently to myself, as I had always found such pain difficult to treat with distal acupuncture. She was my first case of coccyx pain since incorporating bloodletting into my practice.

Her coccyx was not tender to palpation—the pain was deep and she felt it only when making certain movements. It was worst when sitting and when rising from a sitting position. Samantha told me it had been bothering her for over a month, although she did not recall any injury or specific reason for it.

I had never seen a written reference to bleeding for coccyx pain, so wasn't sure how to go about it. In general, the go-to area for bleeding legs is the UB40 area, but Samantha had no visible veins there. She did, however, have just one short, dark vein in her left lateral lower leg, around GB36, which I bled using a 20g hypodermic needle.

When I was done, I had Samantha do the movements that had been causing her pain. She sat in a chair, then stood, then sat, then stood again, then gave me an approving nod and said "Much better—it's not gone completely but much better. Much much better." We made a follow-up appointment for a week later, and she left.

When Samantha came back the next week, she told me she still felt something in her coccyx occasionally but that it really was no longer a problem, and asked if we could work on her shoulder instead.

Teresa's ptosis

Teresa is a 73-year-old artist who paints beautiful landscapes in acrylic. She came to me with several problems, one of which was ptosis in her left eye.

Ptosis is a condition where the upper eyelid droops, partially covering the eye and obstructing vision. In elderly patients such as Teresa, the cause is usually deterioration or stretching of the levator muscle due to aging. The only treatment in conventional medicine is surgery, which Teresa wanted to avoid.

At her first appointment, I bled Teresa's left ear apex for the ptosis and when she left, it was much improved.

But when she came back two weeks later, her left eyelid was again drooping. "It was great while it lasted" she said, "but it didn't last very long. Can you make it last longer?"

Over a period of months, I bled that left ear apex every 2-4 weeks. Each time Teresa got relief. The amount of time the relief lasted would vary from time to time, usually from a few days to a few weeks.

Finally, after perhaps six months of this, the ptosis seemed to stabilize. She still comes in to have it treated, but the relief has become longer-lasting.

Lisa's neck pain

Lisa came in with 2 major complaints—spasms in her upper back and neck, and also right sciatica.

At her first appointment, I palpated her upper back DT.08 and DT.09 areas for tender points and found an extremely tender point at DT.09, which I bled. I also dry-cupped the sore points on her right upper back and neck, and did acupuncture.

The next time she came in, Lisa told me that wet-cupping her upper back had produced a miracle with her sciatica—it was completely gone. But the painful spasms in her neck and upper back were unchanged despite all the acupuncture and dry-cupping I had done.

The fact that Lisa had responded so well to bleeding told me that she was a "blood-stasis type," with a blood-stasis-prone constitution. Her neck and upper back problem had already completely failed to respond to my best dry-cupping and acupuncture. So clearly, the next step was to bleed her.

Where best to bleed for this? The simplest would be to bleed her right ear, but I felt her case warranted a more "heavy-duty" bleeding approach. I could also have bled her right lower back, Master Tung point (or area) DT.16, which is indicated for pain in the upper limbs, shoulder and upper back, or the upper limb zone in her upper back.

But the most likely place to bleed and get the best response was the back of the knee area, the so-called UB40 or occipital region. And that's what I did. The veins she had back there were hard to find but when I finished bleeding them, she had no pain whatsoever.

It's been several months since I last treated Lisa. After her first treatment (where I bled DT.09) her sciatica never returned. Her upper back/neck spasms and pains were more stubborn and did come back, requiring 4 consecutive bleedings every ten days or so to completely resolve, although after the first bleeding they were less painful than at first.

Matthew's varicose veins

Matthew was a 61-year-old man who came to me complaining of pain in the ball of his right foot and toes. He drove for a living, and every time he hit the brake it caused pain.

Matthew was generally healthy, but I noticed he had fairly severe varicose veins in that leg, and asked him about them. He said yes, the varicose veins were a real problem for him as they were not only unsightly, but also caused his legs to ache and feel heavy. He hadn't mentioned them to me because he assumed the only treatment was surgery. It never occurred to him that acupuncture could treat them.

Like most people with varicose veins, Matthew had prominent purple spider veins in his lower leg. I bled the spider veins in hopes of treating both his toe pain and his varicose veins. I also did acupuncture for the toe pain.

A week later he returned for a follow-up appointment and as soon as I saw him in the waiting room, I knew he had had a good result. Matthew was smiling and looked generally very pleased.

"So," I asked confidently, "how's the pain in your foot?"

"The pain in my foot?" he replied. "Oh, it's about the same."

I was puzzled. "So why do you seem so happy?" I asked.

Matthew pulled up his right pant leg and beamed at me. "My varicose veins are almost gone," he said happily. "It's incredible. The achy, heavy feeling is gone too."

I found a few more spider veins and bled them, and told Matthew he didn't need to come back until the symptoms returned. Matthew did come back about a year later for shoulder pain, but the varicose veins were still gone.

Again, the trick to treating varicose veins is to NOT bleed the ropey, green, bulging varicosities themselves. Rather, find the most bleedable dark spider veins in the same leg, and bleed those.

Helen's "stealth" varicose vein treatment

Helen came in wanting acupuncture for high blood pressure. Her very enlightened MD had suggested it, telling Helen that before prescribing anti-hypertensive meds, she would like her to try a course of acupuncture.

Helen had some dark, bleedable-looking veins on her lower leg, so I bled them.

A week later, Helen came back for a follow-up appointment. Her blood pressure was down and her MD was impressed.

But the funny thing was that when Helen came in for her follow-up, the first thing she did was to pull up her pant leg and say "I used to have a varicose vein on this leg and since I was here last week, it seems to have disappeared. Do you think your treatment could have had anything to do with that?"

Why yes ma'am, as a matter of fact I do!!! As I've said many times, one of my favorite indications to do bloodletting for is varicose veins. Works like magic. Just remember to NEVER bleed the ropey varicose veins themselves. Instead, find a dark, flat vein (or veins) and bleed those. More often than not, you will find them on the lower leg, not far from the ankle.

Katie's yearlong foot ordeal

Katie was a 49 year old woman who came into my office on crutches in April of 2014. She had fallen almost a year earlier, and an MRI had revealed a fracture in her right foot.

Her orthopedic doc put her in a boot for 9 weeks, but a follow-up MRI revealed her fracture had not healed. She was put on a bone stimulator 10 hours a day for 6 months, but still that bone would not unite. At some point she also did extensive physical therapy.

Finally, her orthopedic doc gave up and sent her to a pain specialist, who put her on neurontin. That didn't help, so he did nerve blocks on two separate occasions, neither of which gave her relief.

When Katie came to see me, her pain was so severe that it was excruciating to put weight on that right foot, hence the crutches.

The first thing I did was Dr. Tan-style distal acupuncture, which gave her pain relief for a while. But the real breakthrough came when I bled her right Tung point (or area) 11.26, Control dirt. After that, her condition improved rapidly and after a total of 7 visits (during which I bled 11.26 twice), she stopped coming.

In October 2017, more than three years later, Katie came back to see me for an unrelated issue. She could not stop gushing about the miraculous results we had achieved with her foot more than 3 years earlier. I asked if she had ever had a follow-up MRI on that foot to verify that the fracture had healed. "No" she said, "maybe I should, but I haven't had the slightest pain in that foot since I last saw you, so I see no need."

Sheila's heel that wouldn't heal

A case similar to that of Katie (previous case) was that of Sheila A, who had injured her right heel about a year before coming to see me. The heel hurt every time she extended or flexed her foot, which meant pain with every step.

Sheila had also been in a boot for months and had had additional therapies, all to no avail. There was some uncertainty about the exact cause of the pain— one doc looked at her MRI and said there was no fracture, while another said there was.

At her first appointment I just did Tan-style distal acupuncture, which gave her immediate relief. But at her next appointment a week later, Sheila told me she had felt great for 2 days, after which the pain returned as before.

The doctor who saw a fracture in that heel believed it had never healed properly, which would account for its stubbornness. So at her second appointment I bled 11.26, then treated with acupuncture as I had at the first appointment.

This time, at the end of the treatment she said she had NO pain on flexion or extension of that foot, so the pain relief was greater than at the first treatment.

Sheila had just those two treatments, after which I never saw her again. At this writing it is seven months since her last treatment, so I emailed her for an update.

She emailed me back that her experience was great, that "after releasing blood from the thumb" (bleeding 11.26) she felt great relief, that she can now flex her foot well and has no pain when walking. The only remaining issue is an occasional burning sensation on the sides of her ankle and when work lets up, she will come in to address that.

Since Sheila responded so well to bleeding 11.26, my first plan of attack for that ankle will be to bleed the ipsilateral leg—most likely in the UB40 region.

Fay's trigeminal neuralgia

One of my favorite conditions to treat is trigeminal neuralgia. In most cases it responds quickly to bleeding the apex of the ipsilateral ear.

Fay is a 67 year-old woman whose TN began with a tooth cleaning, after which she noticed minor shooting pains on the right side of her face. It got worse and worse over a period of eight weeks, and finally the intense pain became intolerable.

Fay had seen a few dentists and a neurologist, but none of them could offer her relief. To make matters worse, she had sleep apnea and wore a CPAP mask at night, which irritated the painful area.

When she came to me, Fay was experiencing some discomfort all the time, but it was the knife-like attacks of stabbing pain that were making life unbearable. They were unpredictable. On a good day there would be fewer than 5 attacks, but other days the attacks would repeat all day long, as often as every 5 minutes. She described them as "like someone sticking a knife into my nerve." The pain was easily a 10 on a scale of 1-10, and each attack would last about 2 minutes.

At Fay's first appointment I asked her to rate the discomfort she felt at that moment, and she said it was a 2-3 out of 10. I bled her ipsilateral (right) ear apex, and immediately asked if she noticed a difference. She was surprised to note that yes, there was a significant difference, the discomfort had become barely noticeable, perhaps a 1 out of 10

Encouraged by that success, Fay made an appointment for 3 days later. When she came in she reported that the sharp pains were gone, it was now at worst a dull ache, like a toothache in her upper right jaw. I bled her right ear again at a slightly different point than before, and again she reported immediate improvement.

After that, Fay came for treatment every week or two, and the amount of discomfort she felt between treatments dropped to almost zero. After two months of treatment she went on vacation for 4 weeks and when she came back, she reported being almost pain-free the entire time.

After another few months of treatment every 3-5 weeks, Fay came in and said her face was fine, and asked to work on her knee instead. Since then, she rarely feels any discomfort in her face. When she doe,s she comes in promptly for treatment, which keeps her pain-free for many months.

Ben's severe abdominal cramps

Ben was a 54 year old male who presented with debilitating abdominal cramps, which he called an IBS flare-up. He had a history of getting such flare-ups every 1-3 months. He told me the pain was more on the left side, so I bled his left UB40 area.

Before the blood had even stopped flowing, he told me with a stunned look on his face that the pain had disappeared entirely. Since then he has come back twice for the beginnings of a flare-up, at approximately 5-month intervals. Other than that he has been pain-free.

David's hemorrhoids

I haven't had a great many patients come in specifically for hemorrhoid treatment, as most people think that acupuncture involves sticking needles right where it hurts. But in the course of treatment for other complaints, a few patients have told me they have hemorrhoids. In almost every case, bleeding the UB40 area has worked a miracle.

David is a professor of anatomy at a medical school and a longstanding patient who originally came in 6 years ago while recovering from a severe flare-up of Crohn's disease. During his flare-up he was on a high dose of steroids for months, which caused him to develop an anal infection. That turned into an abscess and eventually into a fistula, which required surgery.

The surgery had been successful and had healed completely years earlier, but David was alarmed when one day he developed pain and discomfort in his anus, with bloody stools. He feared a recurrence of his abscess and fistula, but his proctologist told him it was just hemorrhoids. I suggested bleeding his UB40 area, and David agreed.

David was just 42 but had dark spider veins in his popliteal fossa, and I began by piercing one on his left leg with an 18g hypodermic needle. A small amount of dark blood oozed out.

Immediately David—who was lying face down—turned his head and looked at me with a startled expression on his face. "The pressure just came off my anus" he said. "I swear to God, it came off like 90% immediately. Is that possible? Can it really work that quickly?"

I assured him that yes, it can and usually does work that quickly. He could not stop raving about his instant results and as he was leaving, he looked at me and again said "I just can't believe it can work this fast but there's no doubt about it, that pressure is way down. It was instantaneous."

David has been in many times since then for other issues—mostly relating to his Crohn's disease—but has told me whenever I've asked that he never had another symptom of hemorrhoids after that one treatment.

Margaret's endometriosis

Margaret was a 32 year old woman who came to my clinic suffering from endometriosis. This condition typically causes severe pain during menses, with some women suffering even between periods.

Margaret's endometriosis impacted her quality of life as she was one of those who suffered from pain all the time, not just during her periods. Sex was also painful. She had not been able to conceive, and thought that perhaps the endometriosis was the reason. Endometriosis is often associated with infertility.

Margaret had surgery which was successful for a time but, as often happens, the pain returned full-force after six months or so.

At Margaret's first appointment I bled bilateral UB40, one vein in each leg. Immediately the pain dropped from a 5 to a 1 out of 10. I did no other treatment.

When she came for her next appointment a week later, Margaret happily reported that she had had zero pain since the previous treatment. "It was so weird last week how the pain just kind of melted away when you poked my leg with that needle," she told me. "It was just so weird." I bled her again for good measure and sent her home.

A little over a month later, Margaret came back and said she was mostly fine but felt a little pain in her right abdomen during sex. I bled her again and have not seen her since.

Deborah's post-surgical entrapped nerve

A year and a half before coming to see me, Deborah had had emergency surgery for a burst stomach ulcer. Six months later she developed an incisional hernia at the site of the surgery, and had another operation to repair it. The surgeon used Kevlar mesh.

After that surgery, Deborah had severe pain in her left abdomen near (but not at) the incision. Her surgeon assured her that the operation had gone perfectly, and the pain was just post-surgical discomfort that would soon resolve.

But instead of going away the pain worsened. When Deborah came to see me a year after that repair surgery she was virtually incapacitated with "constant horrific pain." A gastroenterologist had ruled out any gastrointestinal cause for the pain. Deborah had seen many other medical specialists but none could find a specific cause for the pain, so finally they diagnosed it as an entrapped nerve due to surgery.

Deborah had seen a pain specialist, who proposed a nerve block. But after looking up the risks, Deborah decided to try acupuncture first.

The first thing I did was Dr. Tan-style acupuncture, but it had no effect. Since her pain seemed nerve-related, I figured bloodletting was my next best bet.

I examined Deborah's left lower leg. I have had success resolving abdominal issues by bleeding legs at various locations, as the choice of where to bleed the leg for abdominal complaints is more a question of bleeding what you see than bleeding specific points or areas. If you find bleedable veins in one or two areas on the leg and in no other areas, bleed those—wherever on the leg they may be. The most common areas to find them are UB40 and the lateral upper half of the lower leg, and also around the ankles.

Deborah had two bleedable veins in her left leg near ST36 and nowhere else, so the obvious choice was to bleed those. I also palpated her abdomen and found one spot that was excruciatingly tender to palpation, so I wet-cupped there, being careful to apply only the most gentle suction.

In retrospect I should have had Deborah give me an update on her pain level after bleeding her left leg—and before bleeding her abdomen—so I would know to what extent each was effective. In any case, after bleeding her abdomen I had her stand and tell me how the abdomen felt. She hesitated for a long time before barely whispering that there was a huge improvement. It was as if—after having suffered crippling pain non-stop for the past year—she was afraid that if she said out loud that it felt better, the pain would come back.

Deborah and her husband have a home in Florida, but whenever she comes back to Chicago she comes in for treatment. It's hard to get her to give me precise numbers such as percent improvement or where she is on a pain scale, but she is always happy and tells me how miserable she was and how happy she now is, and how "I can do everything again." It seems as though she currently has no pain but is afraid to say so out loud. I don't think I've ever had a more satisfied or complimentary patient than Deborah.

Tasha's interstitial cystitis

Tasha is a 39 year old elementary school teacher who came to me with a history of interstitial cystitis, a painful inflammatory condition of the bladder. Until that time, her flareups had tended to resolve fairly quickly. But at the time of her first appointment, Tasha had been suffering from a flareup that was more painful and more long-lasting than previous ones, and had caused her pain continuously for over 3 months.

She was already taking medications but with little effect, and at that point her doctor had nothing to offer other than a procedure called cystoscopy with hydrodistention. This is an invasive and somewhat risky procedure performed in a hospital under general anesthesia, and is done as a sort of "Hail Mary" if less invasive procedures do not work. Possible complications include blood in urine, bladder infection, puncture of bladder wall and worsening of symptoms—not to mention the risks of anesthesia.

Tasha wanted desperately to avoid this procedure, so I bled her bilaterally at approximately ST36. Probably due to the inflammation in her abdomen, the vein was under high pressure, and dark blood spurted for several moments after I pricked the vein. The bleeding was immediately effective however, and the pain reduced some 70%.

That was about three years ago and while I have had to bleed her several times since then, the bloodletting has been able to keep the pain under control. Tasha has gotten immediate relief with almost every bleeding, has been able to reduce the drugs she is taking for IC by a third, and has not needed any additional procedures to control the pain. I alternate bleeding veins in the ST36 area, and veins in the UB40 area. For the past six months she has had no pain whatsoever.

Frank's high blood pressure

Chad is a patient of mine who made appointments for his parents while they were visiting from California. His dad Frank was 64 years old and wanted me to work on his anxiety, arthritis and TMJ.

But in the course of doing Frank's intake, I learned that he had a bigger problem—high blood pressure that could not be controlled with medication. Frank was on two blood pressure drugs and a diuretic, yet his blood pressure still averaged 171/99.

Not every case of hypertension is caused by blood stasis but when it is, blood pressure drugs are of limited effectiveness as they do nothing to resolve the cause. These cases require bloodletting. So whenever I see a case of HBP that is refractory to medication, I am anxious to try bloodletting, which so often produces a miracle.

I had Frank take his pants off so I could examine his entire legs and thighs to see what bleedable veins he might have. In these cases I am looking for the best veins to bleed, and it doesn't matter where on the legs they appear.

Both legs were just white skin except an area of Frank's left lower lateral leg about 3" x 2". There I found 4 fairly large, superficial, dark purple spider veins that looked as though they were begging to be bled. I told Frank what I planned to do. "You're the doc," he replied.

I poked two of the veins with an 18g hypodermic needle. The blood that came out was dark—almost black—but after a while turned bright red. That is an almost unmistakable sign of blood stasis that has resolved, and bodes well for a good outcome. Given that and the fact that his severe hypertension could not be controlled with drugs, I had a good feeling about the treatment.

Frank and his wife came back 3 days later, just before returning to California. He told me that in the 3 days since the previous treatment, his blood pressure had dropped dramatically and over those 3 days had averaged 138/84. Needless to say, he and his wife were delighted.

Recently I bled similar veins in the leg of a patient I was treating for sciatica. At his third appointment this patient asked "Can what you're doing lower blood pressure?" It turned out that he was on blood pressure drugs and had recently noticed that his blood pressure—normally 120/80 with the drugs—had dipped to about 105/73. He was happy about the drop in BP and the prospect of reducing his drugs.

If I know a patient is on blood pressure drugs and I am bleeding him or her for something else, I warn them that they may need to adjust their meds. Most patients are happy to hear that, and even happier if they actually do need to reduce their medication.

One woman I was bleeding for pain, however, was annoyed when she found out her blood pressure had dropped and she would have to make an extra visit to her doctor. But she was thrilled that her spider veins had faded, and so she forgave me.

Lucy's post-mastectomy syndrome

Lucy is a 56-year-old woman who had cancer in her left breast and elected to have a bilateral mastectomy. After the operation, she had bilateral numbness and a feeling of burning on the skin. She said it felt like a severe sunburn, and was so sensitive that it hurt even when touched by her blouse.

The pain was not on the surgical scars; rather, it was several inches above the scars and down her flank. Lucy searched on the internet and found that these exact symptoms are common in mastectomy patients and even have a name—"Post-mastectomy pain syndrome."

The first thing I did was to bleed the apex of both of Lucy's ears, after which she said that she felt much, much better. In fact, the pain and discomfort were virtually gone. I had planned on doing additional acupuncture, but her relief was so complete that I stopped treatment right there and let her go.

At her next appointment a week later, Lucy said the relief had held and asked if she needed to come in at regular intervals or if she could just "play it by ear." I told her that as long as she had no symptoms she did not need to come in, but that she should make an appointment at the first sign that symptoms had returned. That was 3 months ago and I have not heard from her since.

If you look up "Post-mastectomy pain syndrome" on the internet, you will see that it is "a type of neuropathic pain, a complex chronic pain state that is typically associated with nerve fiber injury." Mainstream medicine has no good treatment for it. But in this patient at least, simply bleeding her ear apex one or two times was able to eliminate it, or at least to give her long-term relief.

Lucy's success is another of many examples of various nerve-related pains that have responded to bloodletting.

Jakob's hand and knee

Jakob was a 53-year-old artist who lived in South Africa. While visiting relatives here, he developed severe pain and swelling in his left wrist and hand. His sister, a patient of mine, brought him in for treatment.

Jakob's sister had told me when booking the appointment that he would be returning to South Africa soon, so I made him the last patient of the day as that would give us extra time if necessary. Jakob's left hand and wrist were indeed quite swollen and tender to the touch. He was essentially unable to use that hand.

Jakob told me he got such flare-ups from time to time, and that it seemed to be triggered by stress. There had been no trauma or injury to it. He told me his left knee was in great pain too, and asked if I could work on that as well. I was glad he was the last patient of the day, as I could see we would need extra time.

My first question—to myself at least—was whether or not Jakob was a "blood stasis type." If so, then probably both his hand and knee would respond to bleeding. If not, then in all likelihood I would have to treat him with a different approach. That's not guaranteed—it's possible that one can have one complaint that responds to bleeding, and another complaint that does not. But in the vast majority of cases, blood stasis types have blood stasis problems, and you can count on bloodletting to be effective for most complaints in such patients.

For Jakob's hand problem, the only way to know if was blood stasis would be to bleed him and see if that worked. But for knee pain, simply palpating the DT.07 area in the upper back for a tender point can tell with near-certainty if bloodletting will be successful or not. So that's where I began.

I had Jakob lie face down on the table and palpated his upper left back in the DT.07 area. When I pressed on one point, Jakob visibly flinched and let out a soft grunt. That told me with high confidence I could wet-cup that point and it would greatly relieve his left knee pain. It also suggested that Jakob was a blood-stasis type, meaning that the best treatment for his painful left hand and wrist would probably be bloodletting as well.

I wet-cupped that point in his left DT.07 area, and when I was done I had him stand and test it by walking around. As he did so he smiled and in his soft South African accent told me his knee was "One thousand percent better."

Next I had him lie on his back and bled two veins in the crook of his left elbow, one medial and one very lateral. Again this produced major, immediate improvement, this time in his left wrist and hand. Jakob marvelled at the quick results, as doctors in South Africa had tried many therapies for these flare-ups in his wrist and hand to no avail.

There was just enough time before Jakob's return to South Africa for one more treatment, and he came in the day before his departure. His left knee was free of pain, and the symptoms in his left wrist and hand were nearly resolved. The swelling was gone and Jakob just had some remaining discomfort in his medial left wrist, for which I did a gentle Dr. Tan-style acupuncture treatment, after which Jakob left pain-free.

Rebecca's sciatica

Sciatic pain is something I almost always treat with bloodletting, usually successfully, so choosing a representative case is tough. But Rebecca is a good choice because she has been coming for many years, and also because when she first came to me she was still in pain after 4 surgeries for her right-side back pain and sciatica. She didn't want more surgery, and was ready to try acupuncture as a last-ditch effort to avoid it.

Rebecca had purple spider veins all over her right lower leg, and I would describe those veins as "inviting." In her right UB40 area alone she had prominent purple spider veins—one in the lateral popliteal fossa, one in the medial popliteal fossa, and one in the middle of the popliteal fossa—right at UB40. I bled all three, and when Rebecca got off the table, she told me with great relief that she felt much better—perhaps 70% better.

Rebecca returned a week later and said that the relief she had gotten had lasted, and she wanted to continue and try to get more relief. This time she was wearing shorts, and I saw that on her right lateral upper thigh was the most prominent complex of spider veins of all the ones she had.

The veins there were dark and superficial—perfect for bleeding. Such veins lie just under a thin layer of skin, and so they bleed well with even the most shallow poke of a hypodermic needle. Since they are so near the surface, there is no chance for the blood to extravasate into tissue on its way out of the body, so there is no possibility of bruising. Moreover, bleeding these veins turned out to be highly effective. Rebecca was well aware that she had prominent spider veins there and affectionately called them "my ugly veins."

Over the past few years, a pattern has developed. Rebecca comes in every 8 months or so with a recurrence of sciatic pain and happily declares that "It's time to bleed my ugly veins." I bleed those and her other spider veins, and after a few times, she is out of pain again. Sometimes I also bleed tender points on her right upper back (DT.08 and DT.09) just for good measure.

Sanjay's reflux

Sanjay came in to my clinic complaining of severe acid reflux. He started having the problem some 4 years ago and had endoscopy, which showed esophagitis and Barrett's esophagus. He was taking a high dose of pantoprazole and was careful what he ate—for the last 6 months no alcohol, no coffee, and an overall alkaline diet. But still in the evening his sternum burned. The drug reduced symptoms temporarily, but the discomfort was always there. He was taking one pill in the evening and one in the morning.

I looked at his legs but there was nothing—no visible veins to bleed. So I had him lie prone and palpated along his paraspinals. And indeed he had one very tender point on the right side at about UB21, and on the left side a little lower, UB22. So I wet-cupped them and sent him on his way.

The next day he called and told me it was a miracle, for the first time in 4 years he felt no discomfort whatsoever. What's more, he hadn't taken any drugs since the treatment—he skipped the evening dose and the morning dose as he felt no need, and still he had no symptoms.

At this writing is two months since that treatment, and Sanjay has not felt that reflux in his chest since the first treatment. About 4 weeks after the first treatment he felt acid stomach discomfort, for which I bled him again. Since then he has experienced some gastric discomfort when he eats spicy food, but has rarely needed to take drugs for it.

Greg's upper back pain

When is local bleeding appropriate? The key seems to be palpation. If you can find a local spot with palpation that is markedly more tender than everything around it, this is a good candidate for local bleeding. The main areas for this seem to be the hip at or near the greater trochanter, and the upper back.

A good example is Greg, who came in complaining of pain in his right upper back. It had become so severe it had taken over his life, as it was all he could think of. His upper back was aching and throbbing all the time, 24/7. He'd been to a physician and had imaging done, but nothing was found. He'd been to a chiropractor and done PT, with no result. To put it mildly, he was unhappy and frustrated.

Greg was quick to tell me that he didn't believe in acupuncture. But nobody else had been able to help him, so his wife had convinced him to swallow his pride and give it a try. But he wanted me to know that he didn't expect it to work.

Greg described the pain as diffuse all over his right upper back, but palpation told a different story. When I pressed hard the whole area was tender but there was one point—maybe lateral to UB42 or so—that really made him flinch. It was clearly the focal point of the whole problem.

That was my clue to bleed locally. I wet-cupped that spot and when I was done, I had him sit up and move that shoulder around to see how it felt.

I wish a had a video of the expression on his face. It was a mixture of puzzlement and amusement, as if he was saying to himself "You gotta be kidding me. Don't tell me this stuff actually works!"

I asked him how it felt now. In an upbeat voice he said "Feels pretty good!" and just kept repeating it like he couldn't really believe it, but there it was.

At Greg's second appointment he said it still felt much better, there was just one spot left. I wet-cupped that, after which he said he had no pain at all.

When he came back for his third appointment, however, Greg was unhappy. His back was still a lot better than when he first came in, but he had left my office the previous time with high expectations that he was done, yet the pain in that one spot near UB42 had come back.

This time I bled 3 veins in the UB40 area—medial, lateral and center. I also pricked his ear, and blood virtually poured out—much more than the typical patient. This is not unusual in "blood-stasis-type" patients, and usually a good sign.

When he came for his 4th appointment, Greg was again happy. He could barely feel some faint symptoms near UB42, and that only occasionally. I again bled that spot directly, and again bled his right ear. This time blood came out of his ear normally.

A week later Greg came for his 5th appointment, but he didn't really need it as he said he had no symptoms whatsoever. But since he was there, I again bled UB40 just for "insurance."

I consider Greg to be a "pure blood-stasis" case. Over the course of treatment I never did acupuncture or any other modality on him, only bleeding.

Karen's ankles

Karen is a Crossfit athlete who came in with pain in both ankles. Her best friend was a chiropractor and together they had tried everything imaginable for over two years to make those ankles feel better, but nothing worked.

I tried distal acupuncture first but that didn't work, so I bled her ub40 area. She didn't have much there to bleed—just the faintest green veins.

A week later she came back, this time accompanied by her friend the chiropractor. They were both giddy with excitement because for the first time in the years they'd been working on her ankle pain, she had gotten significant relief. The chiropractor had come to watch me bleed her friend, and as the blood flowed she just kept repeating "This is SO COOL!!!"

Since then, Karen comes back from time to time when her ankles start acting up, specifically demanding bloodletting. She LOVES bloodletting—of all my patients, she is the most crazy about getting bled. As she lies face down she is always filming me as best she can, even though she can't see anything, and I suspect these videos are all over her FB page.

The more I bleed, the happier she is—she is the perfect fit for my practice. I wish all my patients were such bloodletting aficionados.

Marty's cluster headaches

Marty came in to my office looking beaten-down and didn't even want to talk. His wife told me he'd had a severe non-stop headache for the past 4 weeks. The pain had been disabling most of the time. No drug had helped, scans showed no pathology, and his neurologist had just diagnosed him with cluster headaches.

Usually his pain was 8-10/10 and in the left temple. The previous day it had been at the top and back of his head, and a steady 4/10. He was depressed at having to live with the constant pain.

The first thing I did was bleed both ears, which brought the pain down to 3.5/10. That encouraged me to do additional bloodletting, and I bled veins on both lateral legs. That further brought the pain down to 2.5. I then did acupuncture and let him snooze for an hour. When he was leaving I asked what the pain was now. With some enthusiasm he held up his index finger to indicate 1/10. And he actually smiled.

When he came in, Marty was drooping—beaten down and defeated. When he left, he had a spring in his step. I never saw him again.

Liv's painful, swollen arm and hand

Liv was a 47 year old woman who came in with pain in her right arm and excruciating pain in the hand. The arm was also swollen and the hand was REALLY swollen, "puffy" even. The pain in that hand was a 9. This had come on out of nowhere two weeks earlier, for no known reason. She had seen a doc that day, who told her there were no blood clots or anything that required immediate attention, and scheduled x-rays for later that week.

From the start, Liv was skeptical, suspicious, and stand-offish. It was as though she wanted me to help her, but didn't trust anything I did.

It didn't help when I told her I wanted to bleed her right ear. Why? How? What will that do? Does it hurt?

Finally she let me bleed her ear. It barely bled. I was sure she would scowl at me and say it didn't do anything but when she moved her arm and palpated it, she admitted that it felt a little better above the elbow. But nothing had changed from the elbow down.

I looked at the crook of her elbow and she had two visible veins, one medial and one lateral. So I told her the next step was to bleed those. More questions and skepticism. Is it safe? How much blood? But she could see that the ear bleeding had given some relief so she relented and said okay.

I bled the medial and lateral veins and got a modest but adequate amount of blood. After that she said her arm above the elbow was much better, and she now felt some relief halfway down her forearm too. But the right hand was still puffy and just as painful.

I seemed to be bleeding my way down her arm, so next stop was her jing wells, which I bled. But this had no effect, zero change.

She'd already had significant relief and this was her first appointment, so I could have stopped there. But she was the last patient of the day so I had time, and I felt there was still a key point to bleed that was waiting to be found. I didn't want to let her go without at least some relief in that hand.

I looked at her right leg for some clues, but did not see any bleedable veins there. So I had her lie prone and palpated inferior to her clavicle on her scapula, in the upper limb zone. And bingo, I hit one spot in the scapula upper limb zone that made her jump and groan in pain.

So I wet-cupped that point, on the lateral scapula at about T4, and the blood flowed pretty freely. I filled 3 consecutive cups in short order.

When I was done, I had her stand and we both noticed immediately that the swelling in her right hand was way down. It was still bigger than her left hand but that puffy quality was gone; you could now see the bones. The pain in her hand was down too, and now confined to her mid-palm. The arm was much better too. When she left she was smiling and happy and looking forward to her next appointment.

So I would say if it's a blood stasis issue you're working on—i.e. bleeding has worked—but the relief is less than 50%, keep on going, there is probably more you can do.

Scott the dentist's TMJ

Scott is a dentist who came in for severe right-side facial pain. He had diagnosed himself with TMJ and more, as TMJ did not fully account for the amount of pain he was in. The pain was focused just in front of the ear and at the occiput. Not just a dull ache, but really acute pain—so bad he said he was having a hard time concentrating on a root canal he had been doing before he came in.

The first thing I did was to bleed his right ear apex. When I was done he said the pain was down about 30-35%. So now I knew it was a blood stasis issue, which called for more bleeding.

I had Scott lie prone and pulled up his pant leg. He didn't have much in the way of visible veins, the only one I could see was a little one in the medial popliteal fossa. So I bled it.

I then had him come and sit in a recliner for regular acupuncture. At that point he told me his pain was down 90%—almost gone. He could not believe how quick and effective bleeding had been and told me "I am going to send you so many patients... Now I can tell them with total confidence how effective this is."

Veronica's nausea

Veronica is a lovely woman who unfortunately suffers from recurrent cancer. As a result, she gets an infusion of chemotherapy once a week, one of the side-effects of which is severe nausea. She cannot tolerate the anti-nausea drugs she was prescribed, so she asked if I could treat her for it.

At her first appointment, I had Veronica lie face down and bled DT.03, which is the powerful Master Tung bleeding area for nausea. Using 2 McKesson 17g safety lancets, I pricked 2 points on the spine, just above the hairline, pinching up the skin for extra safety. By the time I had cleaned up and Veronica got off the table, she reported that the nausea was gone and she felt great.

This has become our weekly routine—Veronica comes after her chemo treatment and by the time she leaves, her nausea is resolved.

Maria's recurrent kidney infections

Maria is a 47 year-old woman who presented with a history of recurrent kidney infections. It had started a year earlier; after the first round of antibiotics she had remained infection-free for 5 months. Then the infection came back.

Since then the infection had returned multiple times, and each time the interval between ending a round of antibiotics and the return of the infection shortened. After her previous round, she had been symptom-free for just 3 days. The day she came in, she was on day 4 of a round of antibiotics and STILL felt symptoms. Clearly, the situation was getting worse and worse.

Her symptoms included chills, fever, and—most disabling—severe pain in her left flank.

I figured if I could help reduce inflammation in her left kidney, that would ease her symptoms. More importantly it might also improve blood flow, allowing the antibiotics to get where they needed to go, since part of the resistance to antibiotics may have been due to inflammation and the resulting decrease in microcirculation.

But how to markedly reduce kidney inflammation quickly with acupuncture?

The answer, obviously, was bloodletting. But where to bleed for a kidney problem that is both acute and chronic? Weh-Chieh Young, a direct apprentice of Master Tung and a leading authority on Master Tung, recommends above all bleeding the VT.05 area for kidney issues—particularly a point approximately one cun above and lateral to the navel.[19]

I had Maria lie on her back and palpated her abdomen. Amazingly, the exact point Weh-Chieh Young described was the most tender by far—confirming that was the point to bleed. So I explained what I was about to do. I guess it sounded crazy because she looked at me skeptically and said "How long have you been doing this?"

But she agreed to let me do it so I got out 4 McKesson 17g safety lancets, pricked and cupped GENTLY, and got a modest but adequate amount of blood. When I was done I pressed again on that spot and asked if there was any change. "Yes" she said, "it hurts much less." Her flank pain had been a 6 or 7 just before bleeding so I asked how it was now. She hesitated before saying "I don't feel it." "Not at all?" I asked." "No, at the moment I don't feel anything" she said.

When she left she was so happy, she was telling the friend she came in with how great she felt, booked several more sessions, and told her friend she should book some sessions too.

The rest of Maria's case is interesting so I will tell it here: some weeks later she became delirious with fever and her brother and father, both of whom were deceased, "appeared" and told her she needed to have her breast implants removed. She went to Mexico, where she originally had them done, to have that checked out. Sure enough, they were 15 years old and were leaking. She had them removed and felt better immediately, and the fever resolved. I recently spoke to her sister and, more than a year later, Maria is doing fine. After the leaking implants were removed, the kidney problem never returned.

Curt' knees

Curt is a 65 year old auto mechanic who came in with constant pain of 8/10 in both knees, not controllable with pain meds. He had failed every therapy including cortisone shots, Synvisc injections and more, and had been told for the past 20 years he would need knee replacements. He had refused because he believed the subsequent loss of flexibility in his knees and inability to kneel would end his career as a mechanic. He was at the end of his rope with pain, and was hoping acupuncture might give him a few more surgery-free years.

At the first appointment I palpated DT.07 bilaterally on Curt' back, and both sides were INCREDIBLY tender—a good sign. So I wet-cupped bilaterally and got a lot of blood, and Curt got immediate relief. I continued doing the same at every appointment, each about two weeks apart, along with distal needling after bleeding.

There's been a direct correlation between the reduction in tenderness at DT.07 and the reduction in knee pain. After several weeks, Curt' DT.07 points were barely tender—very hard to find—and when I bled them there was not much blood. At the same time, he reported that his pain had been better than ever—a 1/10. He told me his knees felt better than they had in the past 30 years.

Matthew's reflux

Matthew is a 70 year old man who has had digestive problems—most prominently severe acid reflux—his whole life. Almost anything he ate aggravated it, and in the evening it became a major problem, disturbing his sleep almost every night. He had tried every possible drug to no avail; the only thing that helped was a severely restrictive diet during which he ate almost nothing.

At his first appointment I did acupuncture on him, which had no significant effect. At the next appointment I wet-cupped his back at around DT.15. This helped, but not dramatically.

At his third appointment I wanted to bled his legs, but it was hard to find any veins. He had a faint "shadow" running through ST37 or so—so faint I wasn't sure if it was a vein or if I was imagining it. But when I pricked it, dark blood ran out.

This time, the change was dramatic. Matthew had eaten a donut that day which, he told me, is always a disaster, and in fact he came in that day suffering from severe reflux. Normally once that starts, no drug will stop it and it will only go away with time.

But by the time he left my office after bleeding, the reflux was gone and "that never happens. In my whole life, I've never had anything work that quickly."

In the week since that appointment, Matthew felt so good that he ate many things he normally avoids, and even went to a new barbecue place. "Normally that would kill me, I would be up all night. But that night I had no problem."

The lesson to be learned from Matthew's case is that patients don't always need to have dark veins in order for bleeding legs to be effective. Matthew's legs were as free of visible veins as most teenagers. His case is particularly striking in that at 70 years of age, most people have some visible veins even if they don't have an acute blood stasis issue.

Dale's left sciatica and knee

Dale came to my office complaining of sciatica in her left leg. At her first appointment I bled her left UB40 area. She had many veins there and I bled them all. Her pain immediately reduced by some 80%, which is not unusual with sciatica patients.

At her next appointment Dale said she had little sciatica pain left, but there was something else she wondered if I could work on. Her left knee was so painful—and x-rays showed that the cartilage had been so badly destroyed by arthritis—that she had total knee replacement surgery scheduled in 30 days.

Dale hadn't mentioned her knee at the first appointment because she assumed there was nothing acupuncture could do, as she had tried and failed multiple knee therapies including cortisone shots and Synvisc injections. But since the treatment for sciatica had worked so well, was there anything I could do for that knee?

When I asked her how painful the knee was at that moment, she told me 10/10 without hesitation. That was the same knee where I had extensively bled the UB40 area previously. As effective as that had been for the sciatica, it had had no effect on the knee.

I had Dale lie prone and palpated her upper back in the DT.07 area. When I lightly pressed one point, she jumped and yelped in pain. I had barely touched it so I was certain this was the spot to bleed. That was confirmed when I palpated the mirror-image point on her contralateral upper back and it was not painful at all.

After wet-cupping that point, I had Dale stand and tell me how it felt. She could hardly believe how much less it hurt—"If it was a 10 before, it's a 2 now" she said.

At her next appointment, I bled her left DT.07 area again at a tender point just next to where I had bled previously. As she was leaving she told me she had zero pain in that knee and wondered aloud whether to cancel the knee replacement surgery, which was now scheduled to take place in 20 days.

Dale had a few more appointments over the next few weeks. The pain in her knee during that time varied from zero to about 4/10.

In the end however, Dale decided to go ahead with the operation. It was October and she had already reached her $7,500 insurance deductible for that year. If she cancelled it and decided to do it the following year, it might cost her the full $7,500 deductible.

The most interesting thing about Dale's case is how locally bleeding that knee produced no result, while distal bleeding was highly effective. This is not the case every time, but in perhaps 9 out of 10 cases it is—especially pain of degenerative origin such as this. Delia's case—which follows—is the exception to the rule.

Delia's knee

Delia is a young woman who came to me after having injured her right knee skiing a few months earlier. The pain was not great; what bothered her was the constant tightness and discomfort. But the most disconcerting aspect of the injury was the swelling, which was not getting better.

X-rays had shown a tibial bone chip at the knee, which her doctors believed was preventing the swelling from getting better. An MRI would have shown more, but she could not have one due to having metal internally from a previous heart surgery. Her doctors told her she would probably just have to live with the swelling and discomfort, which might or might not resolve with time.

At Delia's first appointment, I had her lie prone and palpated her right DT.07 region on the upper back. I found a point that was marginally more tender to palpation than the surrounding area, and wet-cupped it. I also did distal acupuncture. When she left she said she did not feel any reduction in symptoms, so I suggested we wait a few days and see what developed.

At her next appointment, Delia told me her knee was still no better. Clearly, bleeding DT.07 was not going to be the magic that it usually is for knee problems.

That knee did have some bleedable-looking veins on both the anterior and posterior aspects. Normally I don't bleed knees locally, as doing so rarely produces good results. But in this case, bleeding distally had not worked. Also, the presentation was unusual—tightness, discomfort, and swelling rather than pain.

I had her lie face down and with a 20g hypodermic needle, bled 3 veins in the UB40 zone—lateral, medial and middle. The middle one spurted several inches for a few seconds—an excellent sign that this would probably be effective. And indeed, when she stood and flexed her knee, the discomfort was much reduced.

Delia enjoyed acupuncture treatment and especially enjoyed bleeding, and insisted I bleed her at every appointment. She wanted to come twice a week, so it was challenging to find new veins to bleed each time, as I did not want to bleed the same vein more often than once every ten days or so. I bled the posterior and anterior leg and also the thigh—wherever I could find a bleedable vein. Fortunately she had quite a few.

Delia made rapid progress. After 5 appointments, her swelling was not noticeable and her tightness and discomfort were gone. At this writing, she continues to come weekly for stress relief and to keep working on the knee so the problem does not return. I continue bleeding it from time to time as appropriate, and she is always happiest when I do.

Sarah's blocked axillary sweat glands

Sarah was a 17 year old girl who came in with a history of recurring blocked axillary sweat glands. They would become swollen, painful, hard, and sometimes infected. Her doctor kept surgically excising each new one as it would occur.

Finally, she and her mom decided there had to be a better way, and came in for acupuncture. At her first appointment, she came with a blocked, swollen, left axillary sweat gland. I bled her left ear apex; the next morning she woke up and the sweat gland problem had resolved.

A few months later she came back with the same problem in her right armpit. I bled her right ear apex and two days later the problem in her right armpit was gone.

At this writing—8 months after she first came in—I have had to repeat the treatment for her left armpit one time, which was again effective. Other than that she has had no recurrences in either armpit.

Marci's optic neuritis

An MS patient named Marci came in recently with a flareup of optic neuritis. This is an inflammation of the optic nerve that MS patients are prone to, and it can have serious consequences, including blindness.

In Marci's case her vision, and especially her color perception, was severely affected. It was worse in her right eye, although her left eye was affected as well. She had seen a specialist but all he could offer was a course of steroids, which had not been effective.

The only therapy I did for Marci's eyes at that appointment was to bleed the apex of both ears. Before the blood had stopped flowing and without my even asking, Marci expressed amazement that there had been an immediate, dramatic improvement in her vision, and particularly her color saturation.

After two such sessions, Marci's left eye returned to normal. The right eye returned to normal after three sessions. She came in many months later for a different problem, and reported that her optic neuritis had not returned.

Marci's case is notable in that bleeding her ear apices—a safe, simple, 5-minute procedure performed with two $0.04 diabetic lancets—produced results beyond what the most highly-trained specialist using the most modern and expensive equipment and drugs can achieve.

Bret's son's fever

The following was posted on the Facebook group Chinese Medicine Bloodletting. Used with permission.

My 8 year old son has been sick in bed all day with a garden variety fever. But this one got him pretty bad. He was whining and moaning. In and out of sleep all day and not able to do much else. My wife said he was asking for me all day. He was requesting "Shoni Shin".

When I got home from the office, he woke up and was delirious. He wasn't making any sense. He was HOT! Boiling away. Ear temp said 103. but we all know that's not that accurate.

What he was able to make out was that his head hurt over his left eye.

My wife (who had been caring for him all day and was exhausted) asked what I could do for his headache. I thought "well, I could let his ear apex". So that's what I did.

It spurted out! But stopped relatively quickly. Not even enough to saturate one 4X4.

I was really just hoping to relieve his headache.

She had to hug him tight around his shoulders to restrain him a bit to let me get it done. He was startlingly hot.

Within seconds, my wife was asking is it possible that he's cooler in disbelief. His body cooled down almost instantaneously. Thermometer read 100.7

He became himself almost immediately. No more delirium. Soon after, he asked if he could come downstairs and watch TV. Then he asked for something to eat.

The difference is startling.

Oh, the headache behind the eye is gone too.

Appendix I—Supplies

Single-use safety lancets

- McKesson Safety Lancets 17 gauge (sold under the name "Acti-Lance" outside of North America)
- Capiject 17 gauge safety lancets

21-gauge manual lancets

- I prefer these for bleeding ears. I usually use the brand EZ-lets but any reputable brand should work well

Needles for bleeding veins

- McKesson or BD brands, 18 gauge or 20 gauge, 1.5 inches

Drape paper for the table

- 3-ply McKesson 40" x 72" Drape Sheet. There are many types of table paper and drape sheet available and this is really a personal choice.

Impermeable underpads

- Often sold under the brand name "Chux," I recommend placing these under a limb where you plan on bleeding veins. Probably not necessary when wet-cupping. I currently use Attends Dri-Sorb Underpads 17" x 24"

Disposable single-use plastic cups

- Widely-available and economical disposable plastic cups are made by DongBang company in South Korea. These are available in the US from acudepot.com and kmsupplies.com. Be sure to order a pump

that fits—preferably the pistol-grip type, not the tube-type, for which you need to use two hands which is clumsy.
- You can also order these directly through AliBaba.com, from WorldTech Co. Ltd. Their minimum is 1,000 cups, although that may be negotiable. I have ordered from this company and my order was delivered from Korea to the United States with no problem. I have no association with them.

Roll of plastic bags to put over pump

- The roll I use was ordered through Amazon, (11" x 14" Non-Print 1520 HDPE Grocery Bags).

Hemostatic agents (used to stop bleeding)

- There are so many of these readily available that it is difficult to recommend one brand or type over another. You can buy gauze impregnated with hemostatic powder (hemostatic gauze) in any drugstore, you can also go online and find many such products available such as Quickclot, Celox, and many more.

Gauze (preferably sterile).

- In addition to 2" x 2" and 4" x 4", additional sizes that may be useful are 5" x 9" and 4" gauze rolls

Povidone iodine (Betadine) liquid and/or wipes

- Provides additional disinfection when it's desirable. Be sure to ask patients first if they are allergic to iodine.

Hydrogen peroxide 3%

- Works much better than alcohol for cleaning blood that has dried on skin—I keep some in an "alcohol dispenser" bottle to wet a cotton ball and wipe.

Instant cold packs

- To apply to the back of the neck of patients who have fainted or feel "fainty." Dynarex instant cold packs are readily available and inexpensive. Just squeeze at the arrows; chemicals mix inside, producing instant cold

Bibliography

Young, W., & Dong, J. (2010). *Lectures on Tung's acupuncture: Therapeutic system.* Rowland Heights, CA: American Chinese Medical Culture Center.

Young, W., & Dong, J. (2010). *Lectures on Tung's acupuncture: Points study.* Rowland Heights, CA: American Chinese Medical Culture Center.

Birch, S. and Ida, J. (2010). *Japanese Acupuncture, A Clinical Guide.* Taos, NM: Paradigm Publications

Chuan-Min Wang, (2013). *Introduction to Tung's Acupuncture.* Lombard, IL: Chinese Tung Acupuncture Institute

McCann, H. (2014). *Pricking the Vessels: Bloodletting Therapy in Chinese Medicine.* London UK: Singing Dragon

Zombolas, T. (2009). *Tung Acupuncture: A Quick Reference Guide.* Toronto, Canada

Carson, P. (1988). *Tung's Orthodox Acupuncture.* Taipei, Taiwan: Lien Ho Press Company

Maher, J. *Advanced Tung Style Acupuncture: The Dao Ma Needling Technique of Master Tung Ching-Chang.*

Brett J. Editor, CCAOM. (2016) *CCAOM Clean Needle Technique Manual: 7th Edition.*

World Health Organization. (2010). *WHO guidelines on drawing blood: best practices in phlebotomy.* Geneva, Switzerland: WHO

Endnotes

1. Weh-Chieh Young, *Lectures on Tung's Acupuncture: Points Study* (Rowland Heights, CA, American Chinese Medical Culture Center, 2008), 6-7.

2. McCann, H.,*Pricking the Vessels: Bloodletting Therapy in Chinese Medicine* (London UK, Singing Dragon, 2014), 32-33

3. Salonen, Jukka T., Tomi-Pekka Tuomainen, Riitta Salonen, Timo A. Lakka, and Kristiina Nyyssonen. "Donation of blood is associated with reduced risk of myocardial infarction: the Kuopio Ischaemic Heart Disease Risk Factor Study." American journal of epidemiology 148, no. 5 (1998): 445-451.

4. Holsworth Jr, R. E., Y. I. Cho, J. J. Weidman, G. D. Sloop, and JA St Cyr. "Cardiovascular benefits of phlebotomy: relationship to changes in hemorheological variables." *Perfusion* 29, no. 2 (2014): 102-116.

5. Houschyar, Khosrow S., Rainer Lüdtke, Gustav J. Dobos, Ulrich Kalus, Martina Broecker-Preuss, Thomas Rampp, Benno Brinkhaus, and Andreas Michalsen. "Effects of phlebotomy-induced reduction of body iron stores on metabolic syndrome: results from a randomized clinical trial." *BMC medicine* 10, no. 1 (2012): 54.

6. Weintraub, Lewis R. "Current uses of phlebotomy therapy." *Hospital Practice* 22, no. 6 (1987): 251-256.

7. Higgins, C, Iatrogenic anemia—a downside of blood testing. acutecaretesting.org 2008

8. Smoller B, Kruskall M. Phlebotomy for diagnostic tests in adults. NEJM 1986; 314: 1233-35

9. Wisser D, Ackern K, Knoll E et al. Blood loss for laboratory tests. Clin Chem 2003; 49: 1651-55

10. Hoffbrand AV, Moss P, Pettit JE. Hypochromic anaemias and iron overload. In: Essential Haematology (5th ed) 2006 Blackwell: Oxford

11. Weh-Chieh Young, *Lectures on Tung's Acupuncture: Therapeutic System* (Rowland Heights, CA, American Chinese Medical Culture Center, 2008), 239.

12 Birch, Stephen and Ida, Junko, *Japanese Acupuncture, A Clinical Guide* (Taos, NM, Paradigm Publications, 2010), 214-215

13 Polish, Louis B., Craig N. Shapiro, Frederick Bauer, Phyllis Klotz, Paulette Ginier, Ronald R. Roberto, Harold S. Margolis, and Miriam J. Alter. "Nosocomial transmission of hepatitis B virus associated with the use of a spring-loaded finger-stick device." *New England Journal of Medicine* 326, no. 11 (1992): 721-725.

14 Lanini, Simone, Anna Rosa Garbuglia, Vincenzo Puro, Mariacarmela Solmone, Lorena Martini, William Arcese, Alessandro Nanni Costa et al. "Hospital cluster of HBV infection: molecular evidence of patient-to-patient transmission through lancing device." *PloS one* 7, no. 3 (2012): e33122.

15 Chuan-Min Wang, *Introduction to Tung's Acupuncture* (Lombard, IL, Chinese Tung Acupuncture Institute, 2013), 199-200

16 Ibid, 204

17 Weh-Chieh Young, *Lectures on Tung's Acupuncture: Points Study* (Rowland Heights, CA, American Chinese Medical Culture Center, 2008), 6-7.

18 Johnson, Susan, Seminar "The Ancient Art of Bloodletting," Seattle 2017

19 Weh-Chieh Young, *Lectures on Tung's Acupuncture: Therapeutic System* (Rowland Heights, CA, American Chinese Medical Culture Center, 2008), 239.

Index

A

abdominal conditions and pain, 127, 156, 160, 190, 195, 207, 220
abscesses, 88, 162, 209, 218–19
Acne, 145
acne inversa, 236
Acti-Lance, McKesson safety lancet brand name outside North America, 24, 59, 76, 94, 168, 239
alcohol, 99, 141, 161, 168–69, 201, 226, 240
allergic rhinitis, 161
amenorrhea, 90–91, 194
anemia, 43
angina pectoris, 165, 190
ankle conditions and pain, 187, 217, 228
ankles, 217, 228
   bleeding veins near, 129, 131, 179, 187–88, 195, 220
   bleeding veins near for hypertension, 215
   bleeding veins near for varicose veins, 215
   gout in, 167
ankylosing spondylitis, 146
anticoagulant drugs. *See* blood thinners
anus, 199, 219
anxiety, 26, 31, 145, 200, 222
arm pain/numbness, 145
armpit
   blocked axillary sweat glands in, 145, 236
   risk of axillary vein thrombosis due to mastectomy, 55
arteries, avoiding, 56
arteriosclerosis, 82
artery puncture, what to do in case of, 153
arthritis, 234

Asthma/difficulty breathing, 189
Axillary sweat glands, blocked. *See* armpit, blocked axillary sweat glands in

B

back, bleeding the, 18, 21, 23–25, 71, 79, 84, 94, 99, 106, 108, 117, 134, 149, 173, 185
Barrett's esophagus, 226
basilic vein, 153
bean, drop of blood the size of large is sufficient, 32
Bedwetting, 203
Bell's palsy, 161, 167, 175
Betadine, 49, 74, 168, 201, 240
biological waste, 57
Birch, Stephen, 53
bladder conditions, 90
bleedable-looking veins, 173, 215, 235
bleeding disorders, 41, 53
bleeding needles, 21, 41, 44, 111, 134, 136–37
bleeding regions of Master Tung. *See* regions, bleeding of Master Tung
bleeding the arms (*see also* cubital fossa), 151, 155
bleeding the back, 18, 21, 23–25, 71, 75, 79, 84, 94, 99, 106, 108, 117, 149, 173, 185
bleeding the ears, 17–18, 26–27, 31, 45, 59–61, 69–72, 147–50, 170, 172–77, 179–83, 195, 199–200, 202–3, 206, 227–30
bleeding the legs, 21–24, 111–13, 115–17, 119, 121, 123, 125, 127, 129, 131, 133–37, 139, 141–43, 185, 190
bleeding varicose veins directly, warning against, 55–56
bleeding veins, 19, 21–23, 64, 66, 70, 72, 111–12, 116, 118, 134, 137, 151–53, 185, 187, 239
blood
  amount taken and hemoglobin levels, 43
  amount taken from ear, 60, 147, 149
  amount taken in bloodletting, 22, 31–33, 43, 99, 125, 150, 168
  arterial, 20–21, 56
  dark, 122, 219, 221, 233
  letting just a small amount of, 32, 55, 69, 157, 166, 181, 188

Index

   need to cup to get adequate amount of, 23, 25, 77
   sight of, 71, 134
blood cancer, 36
blood donation, 19, 35–37, 243
blood donation and reduced risk of heart attack, 36–37, 243
blood donors, 36–37, 44
bloodletting, therapeutic, 56
Bloodletting and Western Medicine, 35
blood pressure, 31, 172, 195–96, 208, 215, 222–23
blood pressure drugs, 222–23
blood pressure measurements and axillary lymph node removal, 55
blood stasis, 10, 20, 30, 54, 72, 107, 111, 117, 142–43, 171, 173, 222, 224
   issues caused by, 50, 71–72, 84, 150, 155, 182, 224, 230
   signs of, 20, 171, 222
   spurting blood an indication of, 143–44
   type of patient prone to developing, 29, 173–74, 213, 224, 227
blood stasis constitution, 29
blood thinners, 40, 46, 51–53, 57
blotches, purple, 50
bone, non-union of, 188, 201, 216
bronchitis, 86, 189
bruising, 46, 72–73, 111, 115, 123–24, 141, 151–53, 155, 170, 225
   applying firm pressure to minimize, 40, 46, 52
   informing patients about, 48–49
   in patients on blood thinners, 57
   rarely occurs when bleeding ears, 26
   severe, consequence of failing to apply pressure, 50–52
   unlikely when bleeding dark superficial veins, 47, 52
   unlikely when performing capillary bleeding (wet-cupping), 72

C

Capiject safety lancets, 94, 239
capillary bleeding, 17–19, 21, 23, 25–26, 46, 50–51, 59, 70, 72, 76, 144, 147
   safety of, 51
Cardiac conditions, 189
Cardiovascular benefits of phlebotomy, 36, 243

cardiovascular events, 37
carpal tunnel syndrome, 85, 145
chest conditions, 188
chickenpox and shingles, 170
Chinese Medicine Bloodletting Facebook group, 5, 237
chronic fatigue syndrome, 164
chronic skin ulcers, 162
Chux, 161, 239
Circulatory system conditions, 195
clean field, 99, 137, 149, 168–69
Clean Needle Technique (CNT), 40–41
Clean Needle Technique and bloodletting, 40
Clinical and Laboratory Standards Institute (CLSI), 39
clotting, delayed, 51
clotting time, 33, 52–53
cluster headaches, 228
coccyx pain, 194, 212
cold packs, instant, use of in patients who feel "fainty", 45, 240–41
colds, severe, 88–89
compartment syndrome, 30, 52
Concussion, 201
Conjunctivitis, 145, 172, 176, 210
contraindications, absolute, 53, 55
contraindications and cautions, 49
Control dirt (Tung point 11.26), 162, 187, 216
cosmetic bleeding, 124
cotton
   disposal of blood-soaked, 57, 100
   sterile, 40
   use of vs gauze, 40
cramps, abdominal, 192, 207, 218
Crohn's disease, 218–19
cross-contamination, 14, 24, 59, 61, 76, 94, 96
cubital fossa, 46, 151–53, 155, 175, 181–83, 189, 191

D

D&C, 165

diabetes, 49–50
diabetic lancets, 13, 17–18, 22, 25, 60, 70, 134, 136, 161–62, 176, 202, 237
digestive conditions, 192
disposable cups, 28, 61, 95–96, 167, 169, 201, 211
dysmenorrhea, 194

E

ear
   bleeding, 17–18, 26–27, 31, 45, 59–61, 69–72, 147–50, 170, 172–77, 179–83, 195, 199–200, 202–3, 206, 227–30
   bleeding posterior of, 195
ear conditions, 146, 179
ear region, Tung bleeding zone on legs, 179
ears, massage before bloodletting? 150
emotional upset/psychological disturbance, 200
Endnotes, 243
endometriosis, 190, 194–95, 207, 219
entrapped nerve, post-surgical, 191, 220
esophageal pain, 181
eye conditions, 26, 117, 172, 175, 210
eye protection, 32, 169
EZ-Lets 21 gauge manual lancets, 61

F

Facebook group Chinese Medicine Bloodletting, 5, 237
facial pain. *See* trigeminal neuralgia
faint greenish veins, 137
fainting, 21, 31, 44–46, 73, 111, 124, 126–27, 133–34, 137, 140, 148, 151–52, 233
   history of, 45, 148
favorite conditions to bleed for, my, 175, 178, 185, 187, 190, 195–96, 199–201, 203, 205, 207, 209, 217
finger pain, 183
fingers, arthritic, 201
firm pressure, applying to stop bleeding and bruise formation, 46, 51

Foot pain and numbness, 187
fractures, 188, 215–16
Frontal headaches, 174
Frontal region, Tung bleeding zones on legs/feet, 174

G

gauze, sterile, 39–40, 74, 141, 149, 153, 161, 203
GB14, 176
GB34 area, 207
GB36, 128, 212
GERD. *See* reflux
Glass cups, 77
goggles, wearing when treating shingles, 169, 202. *See also* "eye protection"
goiter, 156–57, 180–81
gout, 167–68, 172, 201, 206
gynecological conditions, 91, 194

H

Hand and finger pain and numbness, 146, 183
Hashimoto's thyroiditis, 180
headaches, 173, 175, 237
  bleeding DT.13 for, 90
  bleeding ears for, 26, 69, 71–72, 145–46
  bleeding legs for, 174
  bleeding pregnant women's ears for, 54
  bleeding Tai yang for, 170, 174
  in children, 237
  frontal, 174
  involving the neck, 175
  occipital, 93, 127, 133, 175
  parietal, 174
  seeing patient during, 174
  side effect of hypertension drugs, 208
  vertex, 174
healing, delayed, 162–63

health inspectors, 39–40
heart attack, reducing risk of, 36
heart attack incidence in blood donors vs non-donors, 36
heel pain/plantar fasciitis, 187
hematomas. *See* bruising
Hemochromatosis, 35
hemoglobin, reduction in due to bloodletting, 43
hemophilia, 53, 57
hemorrhoids, 32, 127, 172, 199, 209, 218–19
hemostasis, 52, 73, 141, 153
hemostatic gauze/products, 33, 51–52, 57, 240
hepatitis, 191
hepatitis B
  microscopic amount of blood sufficient to transmit, 63, 244
  preventing transmission of, 96
hidradenitis, 236
high blood pressure, 31, 146, 170, 172, 195–96, 208, 215, 222–23
hips, 172, 188, 226
hospitals, 28, 39, 43, 65, 134, 136, 221
HTJJ points, 211
Hydrogen peroxide, 141, 240
hyperhidrosis, 146
hypertension. *See* high blood pressure
hypodermic needles, 21–22, 24, 28, 44, 64–65, 111–12, 134, 136–37, 139, 162, 165, 167, 219, 222, 225

I

incisional hernia, 220
inductions, labor, 165
infection, 41, 65, 162, 170, 209, 231
infertility, 195, 219
inflammation, 30, 70, 143, 221, 231, 236
Inflammatory bowel disease (IBD), 91
inflammatory bowel syndrome (IBS), 190
informed consent, 71
injury, 162, 187, 201, 211, 235
  spinal cord, 194, 211

insomnia, 145–46, 200
iodine, povidone (Betadine), 49, 74, 138, 168, 201, 240
itching, severe, 80

J

Japanese bloodletting, 54
Jaw pain, 26, 180. *See also* "TMJ"
jing well points
   bleeding, 10, 54, 60, 161, 167, 175, 195, 202, 229
   bleeding in pregnant women, 54

K

Keratitis, 177
kidney conditions, 90, 160, 192, 208, 231–32
kidneys, inflamed, 190
kidney stones, 193
knee injury (as opposed to arthritis), 84, 235
knee pain, 23, 75, 78, 83–84, 107, 116–17, 150, 173, 185–87, 206, 224, 232
  atypical, 116
knees, when to bleed locally, 235

L

labor, induction of, 165
lancets, 23, 64, 70, 76, 148–49, 161, 165, 168
  higher gauge equals smaller diameter, 148
  inadequate for bleeding legs, 13, 64
  safety, 24, 71, 76
    gauge of, 94, 148
    how many to use, 99
  safety for bleeding VT.01, 156
  safety for bleeding VT.02, 157
  safety for bleeding VT.03, 158
  single insertion only, 41
lancets for bleeding 55.01, 165

Index

lancets for bleeding ears, 149
lancets for bleeding for gout, 168
lancets for bleeding jing well points, 161
lancets for bleeding the back, 76
lancets for capillary bleeding, 23
lawsuits, phlebotomy-related, 152
leg pain and swelling, 84, 183, 185
legs, bleeding, 21–24, 111–13, 115–17, 119, 121, 123, 125, 127, 129, 131, 133–37, 139, 141–43, 185, 190
LI15, 164
liver conditions, 165
Liver/Gall bladder conditions, 191
Lung zone, 86–87, 189
luo vessels, 19
lymphedema, 55
lymph nodes, axillary, 55, 146

M

mania/madness, 200
Manual lancets for bleeding ears, 60, 181, 239
Manual lancets in spring-loaded devices should not be used, 63
Maruyama, Dr. Masao, 54
mastectomy, pain following, 145–46, 223
mastectomy and lymph node removal, 55
Master Tung, 3, 7, 79
  bleeding anterior neck by, 155
  bleeding areas on the back by, 77
  bleeding ears by, 147
  bleeding occipital zone for hemorrhoids, 209
  bleeding of 30-40% of patients by, 10
  bleeding of back points by, 77, 79
  bleeding zones on legs of, 117–21
  bloodletting by, 10, 77
  Chuan-Min Wang direct disciple of, 79
  use of 3-edge needle by, 135
Master Tung ear region, 119, 179
Master Tung frontal region, 179

Master Tung lung region, 189
Master Tung mouth/tooth region, 180
Master Tung occipital region (UB40 region), 117, 133, 174–75, 185
Master Tung point 11.26 "Control Dirt", 162
Master Tung point DT.03, 81, 205, 231
Master Tung point DT.07, 83, 206
Master Tung point VT.05, 231
Master Tung stomach region, 117, 192
Mastitis, 195
McKesson hypodermic needles, 64–65, 134, 239
McKesson safety lancets, 24, 71, 81, 156–57, 161, 164–65, 167–68, 175, 179, 181, 200–201, 205, 211, 231–32, 239
menstruation, irregular, 90
Migraines, 146
  occipital, 128
miscarriages, 54
  incomplete, 165
mounding around puncture site (bruise forming), 40, 153
mouth
  bleeding inside of, 167, 175
  difficulty opening, 180
  points to bleed for sores in, 166, 180, 203
mouth/tooth region, Tung bleeding zone on legs, 178, 180
multiple sclerosis, 236
myocardial infarction, acute, 36

N

nausea and vomiting, 54, 81–82, 172, 199–200, 205, 231
neck pain, 26, 146, 180–81
Needles for bleeding veins (*see also* hypodermic needles), 64, 239
needle-shy patients, 24, 76
needlestick, accidental, 24, 41, 44, 76, 94
nerve
  optic, 236
  pinched, 145, 172
  trigeminal, 206
nerve damage, 52, 152

nerve pain, 26, 29, 85
  abdominal, severe non-stop, 190
neurological reflex, 31
nosebleeds, 93, 179
nose conditions, 179
numbness, 82, 84–85, 182–84, 187
numbness and pain in foot, 187
numbness and pain in lower limbs, bleeding DT.08 for, 84, 184
numbness and pain in shoulder and arm, 182
numbness and pain in upper limbs, bleeding upper limb zone on back for, 85
numbness of hands and feet, bleeding DT.05 for, 82

O

occipital headaches, 93, 127, 133, 175
occipital zone, Tung bleeding region on legs, 128, 133, 185, 214
optic neuritis, 26, 29, 117, 146, 172, 176, 210, 236
osteoarthritis, 83, 117
Otitis media, 179

P

pain
  coccyx, 194, 212
  dental, 145, 178
  foot, 187–88, 201
  hip, 188
  nerve-related, 223
  neuropathic, 223
  sciatic, 225
  stabbing, 87, 217
  wrist, 182
pain/discomfort, post-surgical, 146
Palpitations, 146
paraspinals, 174–75, 194, 212, 226
parietal headaches, 174
patients, dark-skinned, difficulty of finding veins in, 67

pharyngitis, 146, 181
phlebotomists, 21, 32, 39, 44, 56, 152–53
phlebotomy, 35–37, 39, 43, 45, 134, 141, 152, 182, 242–43
Phlebotomy and metabolic syndrome, 37
phlebotomy guidelines, 39, 141
piercing needles, 64–65, 134–36
placenta, retention of, 165
plantar fasciitis/heel pain, 187
plastic bags, 57, 96–97, 99, 168–69
plastic cups, disposable, 14, 61, 169, 202, 239
plum blossom, 202, 209
Poison ivy/poison oak, 80, 199
polycythemia vera, 35–37
popliteal fossa, 219, 225
position, standing, danger of bloodletting in, 134
post-herpetic neuralgia, 169, 202, 209
post-mastectomy pain syndrome, 146, 223
Post-surgical pain/pinched nerve, 191
pregnancy, bloodletting during, 53–55, 165
pressure
  applying, 33, 60, 73, 141, 149, 153
  applying to stop arterial bleeding, 20, 56
  applying to stop hematomas from forming, 50, 57
  applying to stop venous bleeding, 51, 57
  how long to apply, 48
  how long to apply with patients on blood thinners, 52
  sterility of cotton or gauze used to apply, 40
  tissue, 30
  venous, 30, 143
pressure bandage, 20
ptosis, 26, 29, 117, 146, 172, 176, 210, 213
PTSD, 200
puncture depth of safety lancets, 18
purpura, 50, 53

Q

q-tip, 60, 149–50, 161

R

radiating pain, 29, 85, 172, 187
rash, itching, 80
reactions, neurological, 31
reflux (GERD), 190, 208, 226, 233
regions, bleeding of Master Tung, 77, 118–21, 174, 179–83, 189, 191, 194–95, 235
reproductive issues, 90
respiratory problems, 45, 86
Ribcage pain, 146
rosacea, 94, 161, 179

S

safety lancets, spring-loaded single-use, 25, 63, 77, 96, 112, 162, 168
scarlet fever, 83, 157
schizophrenia, 170, 200
SCI (spinal cord injury), 194, 211
sciatica, 13–14, 29, 55, 84–85, 108, 127, 172, 183, 185, 187, 206, 213–14, 222, 225, 233–34
shingles, 169–70, 172, 202–3, 209
shoulder, 50, 92, 212, 214, 227, 237
  frozen, 151
Shoulder and arm, pain and numbness of, 146, 182, 215
SI10, 85
silicone, medical, 64–65, 134
sinusitis, chronic, 179
skin conditions, 199
smelling salts (no longer recommended for patients who faint), 45
sore throat, 156
SP9 area, visible veins in, 199
spasms, upper back/neck, 214
spider veins, 13, 22, 196, 198, 214–15, 219, 223, 225
  bleeding in legs of pregnant women for varicose veins, 55
spinal cord injury (SCI), 194, 211
sprain, acute low back, 87

sterile
  cotton and gauze need not be, 40
  disposable cups come packaged, 28
  does gauze or cotton need to be? 141
  do protective gloves need to be? 40
  meaning of, 28
  verifying that piercing needles are, 135
  which tools and instruments need to be? 39
sterile aspects of phlebotomy, 39, 141
sterile gauze pads, 141, 170
  large, 203
sterility
  certification of for needles, 65
  of hypodermic needles, 64
  of hypodermic needles vs piercing needles, 136
  of piercing needles may be compromised, 65, 135
stomach region, Tung bleeding zone on legs, 192
stroke, 161, 170, 195, 208
stye, 26, 117, 146, 176, 210
subcutaneous bleeding/hemorrhage, 46, 49, 51–53, 57, 152–53
superficial veins, 30, 47, 52–53, 70
sweat glands, blocked (hidradenitis), 236
Sweaty palms, 146
swelling, 56, 116, 180, 183, 224–25, 230, 235
Synvisc injections, bleeding DT.07 after failing, 206, 232, 234

T

Tai yang, 170, 174, 200
temporal arteritis, 176, 210
therapeutic phlebotomy, 35–37
three-edge needles, 10, 60, 66, 77, 94, 135
throat conditions, 180–81
Throat Moth, 156
thyroid issues, 156–57, 181
TMJ, 146, 222, 230
tonsillitis, 146, 156–57, 181
toothaches, 26, 170, 180, 217

toxins, 80
transilluminators, 66
trigeminal neuralgia, 26, 29, 145–46, 170, 172, 177–78, 206, 217
Tung bleeding regions, 77, 118, 174, 179–83, 189, 191, 194–95, 235
Tung's Acupuncture, 79–80, 242–44

U

UB12, 83
UB13, 83
UB14, 83
UB17, 191–92
UB18, 93, 179
UB20, 94
UB21, 94, 179, 226
UB22, 226
UB23, 191–92
UB40, 10, 140, 185, 187, 200, 214, 220, 225
  position for bleeding, 45
UB40 area, 32, 172, 174–75, 181, 183–85, 190–91, 195, 199, 207, 209, 212, 218–19, 222, 227–28, 234
UB40 region, 181–83, 187, 189–92, 194, 217
UB40 zone, 235
UB41, 83
UB43, 83
ulcer, non-healing, 201
ulcers, chronic non-healing, 201
upper limb conditions, 85, 92, 182
upper limbs, 26, 85, 92, 145, 151, 182, 214
upper limb zone, 85–86, 182–83, 214, 229
Upper Lip (point Shang Chun), 166
Uterine fibroids, 195

V

vaginal discharge, 91
varicose veins, 131–32
  bloodletting for in pregnant women, 54–55

diseased valves in, 130
  effectiveness of bloodletting for, 172, 208, 215
  example of, 55, 196–98
  example of protruding veins that are not, 115, 122, 124
  how to treat, 56, 115, 130, 196, 198, 208, 214–15
  similarity to hemorrhoids, 199, 209
  warning against bleeding directly, 55, 114–15, 196, 209
vasovagal syncope, 31, 44–45, 133
vein finders, 66
Veinlite, 67
veins
  dark, 19, 21, 32, 111, 117, 123, 125, 133, 137, 143, 208, 212, 233
  hard-to-see, 66
  ideal to bleed, 21, 111–12
  prominent, 23, 117–18, 178, 183
  visible, 17–19, 21, 23–25, 75, 77, 111–13, 128, 130, 170, 174–75, 179–83, 187–95, 199, 229–30, 233
veins to bleed and veins to avoid, 122, 185
Venoscope II, 66
venous system, deep, 30
Ventral Trunk points to bleed. *See* VT
Vertex headaches, 174
vision loss due to temporal arteritis, 176
vomiting and nausea, 81, 199
VT (Ventral Trunk) points to bleed, 155–60, 180–82, 192–93, 231

W

Wang, Chuan-Min, 3, 79–80, 242, 244
wet-cupping, 17–19, 24–25, 28, 57, 59–62, 75–76, 94–96, 168–69, 172–73, 188, 202, 209, 212–13, 234, 239
WHO (World Health Organization), 39, 57, 242
World Health Organization. *See* WHO
wounds
  chronic non-healing, 162, 201
  infected, 162
WoundSeal Powder, 57
wrist conditions, 85, 167, 224–25

Y

Yin tang, 174, 179
Young, Weh-Chieh, 7, 46, 147, 231, 243–44

Z

zones, bloodletting, 75, 78–79, 81, 88–93, 117, 159, 172–73, 179

Printed in Great Britain
by Amazon